To Bobby,

part of my life as a friend, husband, and father to our sons.

Our love will always continue to grow as it has for almost 50 years.

To Gail, Judy, and Margie.

Keep old friends but make new ones.

Thanks to all of you for the influence you have had on my life,

Eugenia M. Fulcher

To Dave,

my strength, my love, and my life

and

To Friendship,

Genie, friends forever

Margaret S. Frazier

Preface

Welcome to *Introduction to Intravenous Therapy for Health Professionals*. We hope this text provides you with basic knowledge to safely and precisely administer intravenous (IV) fluids and medications within your scope of practice. We have drawn from our combined years of nursing and medical assisting experiences to give you the information necessary to successfully perform the techniques for IV procedures.

We designed this text to approach IV administration in an easily understandable and interesting format. The text assumes the student has been taught basic sterile techniques and has a basic knowledge of anatomy and physiology, pharmacology and dosage calculations, although a short review is included. The student should also be aware of the statutes regarding the administration of IV fluids in his or her state of practice, as well as OSHA regulations for performing this procedure. Furthermore, you and your instructor should know the professional person who is responsible for your actions as a technician, whether this is a registered nurse, a physician, or a dentist.

In the current health care setting, more nurses, medical assistants, and other allied health professionals are expected to have a basic working knowledge of IV principles and techniques. This textbook provides key information in a clear, concise manner so that allied health professionals will avoid administering medications erroneously, which could result in a liability to the medical practice.

The following text features will make the topic of IV therapy principles and techniques easier to understand and reinforce the learning experience:

- **Chapter Outline** presents the major topics that will be discussed in each chapter.
- **Learning Objectives** alert you to the skills or knowledge you should gain from each chapter.
- **Key terms** introduce you to words or concepts that may not be familiar to you.
- **Basic review of anatomy and physiology** provides a basic understanding of how IV therapy can interact with the body systems.
- Examples of physician's orders and **learning notes** to enhance review of dosage calculations.
- Step-by-step **bulleted lists** provide an easy-to-follow format for learning the IV infusion process.
- End-of-chapter **Review Questions** test your knowledge of the chapter content.
- **Competency check sheets** are provided in Appendix B. These outline standards for performance should meet competency-based education requirements and be used for determining the achievement of competency of the task.

As you work your way through this text, keep in mind that the skills you gain now will make you a better prepared professional in IV techniques in the health care setting.

Acknowledgments

Patient safety and comfort are important elements in patient care. For the medical professional, the level of knowledge that provides TLC while providing a level of care that shows professionalism and trust is of utmost importance. As the field of patient care changes rapidly, the expectations for the health care professional also change. The level of the care provided is only as strong as the knowledge base and the attitude of the person tending to the patient. Because IV therapy has become more commonplace in both inpatient and ambulatory settings, the need for knowledge has rapidly changed. With the change of equipment and supplies, patients are receiving this therapy in more and more settings. This text is intended to provide the basic knowledge of the necessary skills for safety and, with the least pain, provide IV therapy. We are aware that this is only an introductory text and the student should continually keep current as the field changes. Just taking the course without the practice necessary will not make a competent professional in the field. As medications continuously change and the indications for the medications change, the professional must continue to learn the drugs and the indications and side effects for patient safety.

A special thanks goes to Andrew Allen, Publishing Director at Elsevier, who first listened to our ideas for this text and gave us the initial support. To Michael Ledbetter, Publisher, and Susan Cole, Executive Editor, we say thanks for all of your support. A special thanks to Celeste Clingan, Developmental Editor, who took our thoughts and listened and then provided guidance along the way. Without Celeste, this would never have come to fruition. To all of you at Elsevier, thanks for a job well done. You are the greatest group with which to work.

We hope this text will provide the basic knowledge needed to provide good patient care in the practice of IV therapy. To all of you who use the text, we hope that you glean those areas that we have provided, but that you will continue to show TLC to all of your patients who require IV therapy. The patient is the person of utmost importance, and we desire the best for each.

To all who have encouraged us on this journey, thank you, and to our husbands who have missed us at times, special thanks for being patient. We love all of you.

Genie and Margie

Contents

Appendices

Introduction to Intravenous Therapy

Chapter Outline

Brief History of Intravenous Therapy

Reasons for IV Therapy

Cultural Beliefs Regarding IV Therapy

Roles and Responsibilities in IV Therapy
  Administration

Risk Management and Patient Care with Infusion
  Therapy

Patient Care Related to IV Therapy

Learning Objectives

Upon successful completion of this chapter, the student will be able to:

- Provide information of the evolution of IV therapy
- Identify reasons for performing IV therapy
- Evaluate the cultural beliefs of patients regarding IV therapy
- Define the legal and ethical issues related to IV therapy

- Identify those professionals who may initiate and monitor IV therapy and the roles and responsibilities of those people
- Describe patient care needed in IV therapy

Key Terms

chemotherapeutic—agent that provides chemotherapy.

chemotherapy—use of a chemical to treat disease, usually cancer.

colloid solutions—contain protein or starch molecules that are found in extracellular space, such as albumin and dextran. These solutions draw fluid from plasma in vascular space to increase intravascular volume.

crystalloid solutions— contain materials capable of forming crystals in the solution, such as dextrose.

crystalloids—solutes that dissolve in a solution and cannot be distinguished in the solution.

cytoxic—medication that acts as a toxin to cells, normal as well as abnormal.

homeostasis—balance of the internal environment of the body through feedback and responses when faced with external and internal changes.

intravenous—into a vein.

intravenous therapy— administration of fluids, nutritional support, and transfusion therapy into the circulatory system via a vein.

maintenance therapy — IV therapy that provides the necessary daily needs of nutrients, such as water, electrolytes, and nutrition.

osmolality—ionic concentration of a solution or the concentration of dissolved substances per unit of solvent.

peripherally inserted central venous catheter (PICC)—long catheter made of soft, flexible material that is inserted into one of the superficial peripheral veins with the tip located in the superior vena cava.

replacement therapy—IV therapy that replaces deficiencies in body substances by administering natural or synthetic substitutes.

restorative therapy—IV therapy that provides the daily restoration of vital fluids and electrolytes.

BRIEF HISTORY OF INTRAVENOUS THERAPY

Intravenous (IV) therapy includes the administration of fluids, nutritional support, and transfusion therapy. When IV therapy is discussed, the concept is seen as a fairly new practice in the medical field, but the actual use of IV therapy first began in the 17th century with experiments of using blood transfusions to treat illnesses. With the discovery of the circulation of blood by Sir William Harvey in 1616 and the production of the first hypodermic needle in 1660 by Sir Christopher Wren, the field of IV therapy first experimented with injecting substances such as wine and opium directly into the bloodstream through a vein using a quill and bladder. The experiments were banned, and the next use of therapy was in the early 19th century, when blood was used for transfusions for women who were hemorrhaging after childbirth. During the early 19th century, Ignaz Semmellweis had found the first infection-control procedure of washing hands and Louis Pasteur had started studying his germ theory. With these findings, the edict to ban the injection of substances into circulation was raised and the applications of the practice again became an interest in the medical field.

The earliest fluids used for IV therapy that were considered to be safest were infusions of 0.9% of sodium chloride because these were in isotonic relationship to blood. When Florence Seibert found that pyrogen substances were found in distilled water, researchers worked to eliminate these bacteria; as a result, IV fluids became much safer and were more widely accepted.

In 1925, dextrose had been added to fluids to provide a source of calories. However, IV therapy was only used for the most critically ill patients in hospital settings.

In the mid-1950s, two main indications for IV therapy existed—surgery and dehydration—with fewer than 20% of hospital patients receiving IV therapy. The site most frequently used to administer the solutions of dextrose 5% in water (D-5-W) or in 0.9% normal saline (D-5-NS) was the antecubital vein of the elbow. The solutions were allowed to run for 3 to 4 hours and then were discontinued at night. The needle was a 16- to 18-gauge reusable needle, and the arm was restrained with leather straps and a flat padded board. Later in the decade the first disposable plastic sets were available but not widely used. The frequent infiltrations with this equipment led to the introduction of a plastic catheter within the lumen of the needle that allowed the needle to be removed; the fluids were inserted through the flexible plastic cannula inserted in the vein. The insertion of a flexible cannula led to less tissue injury and more comfort, as well as more mobility for the patient.

During the 1960s, fluids were refined so the choice now consisted of approximately 200 different types available for treatment; the field of IV therapy accelerated. Added to the field were piggyback medications, filters, and electronic infusion devices that made IV infusions safer and therefore more commonly used. Medications have been added to the basic fluids for patients who are critically ill, but the availability of medications prepared solely for IV use increased in the last half of the 20th century. Today many drugs are available that may only be administered through a vein, especially in the area of **chemotherapy**. In the 1980s the field further expanded with the use of central venous access for total parenteral nutrition (TPN) and **chemotherapeutic (cytoxic)** therapy.

After experimentation in the early 20th century, fat elements, such as cottonseed oil, were added to the fluids for nutritional support, but were removed from the market by the FDA to protect patient safety because refinement of the fluids and the additives for IV use was necessary. Not until the 1980s did the U.S. Food and Drug Administration (FDA) reverse its ban on fat emulsions of soybean and safflower oil emulsions for IV administration to provide total nutrition for the ill. This advance—as well as the insertion of the **peripherally inserted central venous catheter (PICC)**—expanded the field to allow management of patients who need long-term IV therapy for treatment of diseases or the related symptoms such as pain or mutation.

In transfusion therapy, World War II was an important time with the use of blood and blood products on the battlefields to save the lives of wounded troops. plasma was the first separated blood product to be used, so equipment to separate the blood had been developed. Later in the war, red cells from the separated blood products were transfused to provide additional support for wounded soldiers. Although this text will not discuss transfusion, this is of interest because of the advances this made in surgical procedures and life-saving techniques.

Today the field of IV therapy can be very technical and specialized, with approximately 90% of all patients receiving IV therapy during a hospital stay. But more importantly, this therapy is not limited to the hospital setting today but is occurring in the home, in skilled nursing facilities, and in physicians' offices. The advances in the field of IV therapy over the past 75 years have been enormous, and with the use of this therapy with so many patients in so many settings one would think that infusion therapy will continue to increase during the 21st century.

REASONS FOR IV THERAPY

The goals of IV therapy are to maintain or restore normal fluid volume and electrolyte balance for **homeostasis** and to provide a means of quickly and efficiently administering medications. The IV route may also be used for nutritional therapy or supplements that contain amino acids and other nutrients needed by the body for the building of tissue because solutions containing dextrose only contain sufficient carbohydrates to minimize tissue breakdown and starvation. The type of fluid prescribed depends on the patient's state of homeostasis, the need for nutrition, or both. Maintenance and replacement therapy determinants include the amount of fluid that has been lost, the **osmolality** of serum, serum electrolytes, and acid–base balance of the patient. The physician will decide on the type of fluids depending on these factors and the desired effects from the fluids.

Indications for IV Therapy

For medications to be effective, the active ingredient must reach the bloodstream for distribution throughout the body. Oral medications are absorbed in the digestive tract, and parenteral medications, other than those given intravenously, are absorbed by crossing tissue barriers with a loss in the potency of the medication due to breakdown for absorption. With IV therapy, these barriers do not exist and the entire amount of the medication is distributed through the bloodstream to the body immediately following the administration. Therefore IV medications are effective more rapidly and the amount of medication absorbed closely equals the amount of medication administered. In some instances, such as the brain, some barriers to the medication do occur.

IV routes are indicated for patients who are unable to take medications or sustenance by mouth or for medications that may cause detrimental effects to tissues if given by other than parenteral means, such as chemotherapeutic agents. When drugs are ordered that are altered in the gastrointestinal tract, injectable routes of administration—and perhaps more specifically, IV administration—may be used. For the patient who is unconscious, is unable to swallow, is vomiting, or has other difficulties with skin diseases or gastrointestinal conditions, IV medications may be used. When rapid distribution of medications throughout the body is needed, placing the drug directly into the bloodstream by IV administration facilitates the distribution throughout the body and increases the absorption rate.

Most rationales for providing IV therapy are divided into three categories: maintenance therapy, replacement therapy, and restoration therapy. Each type of therapy has a direct influence and a specific rationale for the type of IV fluids ordered by the physician.

Maintenance therapy provides the necessary nutrients to meet the daily needs of water, electrolytes, and nutritional replacement. The volume of fluids to be infused depends on several factors such as the patient's age, height, weight, physical condition, and amount of body fat. Maintenance therapy is used for patients who have either no intake of fluids by mouth or a very limited volume of oral intake, thus requiring the supplementation of fluids and nutritional elements. This is most frequently seen in inpatient and home health care settings.

When a patient has been deficit in fluids and electrolytes over a period of time, usually 48 hours or more, **replacement therapy** may be needed. Patient indications include nausea and vomiting, diarrhea, starvation, and hemorrhage. Before replacement fluids are instituted, the kidney function of the patient should be assessed so that adequate excretion of fluids can take place. Because of the inherent loss of potassium through excretion, potassium replacement may also be necessary to maintain homeostasis. This type of therapy is often seen in ambulatory care and in home health care settings.

Restorative therapy is the daily restoration of vital fluids and electrolytes. With this indication for therapy, the fluids used are physiologically the same as the fluids being lost as determined by laboratory testing. Often several types of fluids are ordered for administration during the same day. This type of therapy is most often seen in inpatient settings because of the dangers of fluid overload and the need for laboratory testing to indicate the elements for necessary restoration.

The health professional responsible for providing IV therapy to patients, whether in an ambulatory care setting, a home setting, or inpatient care, must be careful to monitor the patient for signs of fluid overload or toxicity. The signs and symptoms may include elevated blood pressure; breathing difficulties; chest discomfort; and other common symptoms of adverse reactions such as itching, rashes, and unusual edema.

Indications for Infusion Therapy

IV therapy also includes the infusion of blood and blood products to replace those lost through hemorrhage or other body functions. Blood is the body "organ" responsible for transport of oxygen and other nutrients to the body tissues and the removal of waste products and carbon dioxide. Blood is unique in its actions and is essential in the sustenance of life. When the blood levels, including those of certain components of whole blood, are reduced, the physician may prescribe the use of infusion therapy to supply the needed components to maintain homeostasis.

Whole blood is composed of red blood cells (RBCs), plasma, white blood cells (WBCs), and platelets. For each 500 mL of blood, 200 mL are blood cells and 300 mL contain plasma. The use of whole blood in treatment of symptoms is not the preferred treatment and is seldom used today; rather, the blood is separated into fresh frozen plasma (FFP), packed RBCs (or packed cells), and platelets. By separating the blood components and supplying the patient with only those needed, the patient is not exposed to unnecessary portions and the valuable resources may be used for several patients. Also, the unneeded components will not overload the body and cause the potential for detrimental effects on homeostasis of the body.

RBCs are used to improve the oxygen-carrying capacity for patients with symptomatic anemia who have not shown improvement through nutrition, drug therapy, or the treatment of the disease process underlying the anemia. The transfusion criteria are based on several variables including hemoglobin and hematocrit levels, symptoms, the reason for the anemia, amount and time involved with the blood loss, and the surgical procedure involved (if any). The transfusion of the red blood cells would be used when operative procedures have a blood loss of 1200 mL or more, whereas **colloid** expanders, such as albumin and dextran, or **crystalloid solutions**, such as lactated Ringer's with dextrose, may be used for blood losses of 1000 to 1200 mL.

Platelets are used to control or prevent bleeding from platelet deficiencies or when the patient has functionally abnormal platelets. Platelet products may be from random-donor or from single-donor units. Indications include hemorrhage, surgery, patients who are not bleeding but have rapidly dropping platelet counts, and patients undergoing chemotherapy.

Fresh frozen plasma is used primarily to replace lost coagulation factors. The plasma is separated from whole blood within 8 hours of collection and may be stored for up to 1 year at −18° or for 7 years at −65°. Indications include patients with multiple coagulation factor deficiencies as a result of liver disease, disseminated intravascular coagulation (DIC), or other coagulation anomalies.

The types of IV fluids are numerous and their uses are extensive, including the use of blood products for treatment of patient symptoms. The physician has the responsibility of assessing the patient needs and ordering the proper IV therapy; the individual administering the therapy has certain responsibilities for patient safety as well, such as monitoring the patient, checking orders for correctness, and calculating the administration rates.

CULTURAL BELIEFS REGARDING IV THERAPY

As with most areas in the medical field, the cultural beliefs, including religious customs, of the patient will affect the way the need for IV therapy is accepted. How the patient reacts to IV therapy will depend on one's cultural perspective, the tenets of these lifestyles, and, in some cases, one's religious beliefs. Unique cultural and spiritual beliefs are the basis of one's perception of judgment, behavior, and self-understanding. These beliefs are dynamic and cannot be ignored when providing medical care because these are the basis for how the patient feels about health and disease and his or her treatment. The cultural backgrounds may even include areas that are detrimental to traditional medical care.

The person administering IV therapy needs a basic understanding of the patient's culture and must not stereotype patients by cultures or religions because each person is an individual with individual understanding of traditional and nontraditional medical care. However, the health professional must be aware of the cultural and religious beliefs that will affect the medical treatment through IV therapy and must be sensitive to those who are not of the same culture as the health professional. These cultural thoughts are even so basic as the way the patient views health and disease. The health care worker's cultural background also has a distinct influence on the acceptance or rejection of IV therapy by the patient. The health care worker must take all measures possible to separate his or her beliefs and influence on the patient's health care needs. This separation is necessary to provide the patient with as unbiased care as possible.

The assessment of the patient, including beliefs and cultural practices, is an important factor in obtaining trust and in providing competent care. Through the assessment, risky behaviors of the patient may be uncovered and handled without causing further harm to the patient receiving IV therapy. Observation of the patient and the use of verbal and nonverbal communication skills are important factors for the health professional. Using these skills will also provide much basic information about how the patient feels about the treatment being provided. Be aware of eye contact and the feelings of modesty and inappropriate touch as the patient provides communication of these cultural differences. Also be aware of family reactions to any medical care. Often the family is the turning point in how the patient either accepts or denies ordered medical care. The time for patient assessment also gives the chance to ask questions of the patient and to answer any concerns he or she may have.

Establish the spirituality of the patient and the beliefs of that religion on IV administration. Always remember that some religions have strong beliefs about any medical care and especially about IV therapy. Be aware that some religious and cultural beliefs have folk healers that may have been used prior to the visitation to the medical professional and these may affect the traditional medical care, and even patient safety.

The health care professional must look at each patient as a whole person and must provide holistic health care for patient safety and professional trust when medical treatment is provided. Cultural and spirituality differences need to be considered when providing IV therapy, and the necessary adaptations must be taken as appropriate. Remember that when the cultural and religious beliefs and the medical practices are in conflict, the health professional has the responsibility to try to coordinate the cultural practices with the medical regimen that has been ordered to provide acceptable patient care for all persons involved.

ROLES AND RESPONSIBILITIES IN IV THERAPY ADMINISTRATION

The role of the person administering IV therapy basically is limited by the medical practices act of the state of practice. Who may be involved in preparing and administering intravenous fluids or transfusions will vary from state to state, and

the health care professional is responsible for knowing and adhering to the laws of that state. As the states change the role of health professionals in the care of patients, including in the administration of IV therapy, the responsibilities for the health care professional also change. Who may or may not initiate or manage the fluids after initiation may change rapidly because the medical field itself is a fluid area. Therefore constant learning and building of a knowledge base as well as staying abreast of the changes in the statutes of the state of practice are essential.

With the role of health care professional initiating IV therapy comes a responsibility to perform the task in a manner safe for the patient receiving the fluids and for the person performing the task. The person who is either initiating or monitoring the therapy has legal and ethical practices that are indicated by what is considered the standard of practice for that profession. The legal issue may be a tort that is as simple as starting fluids for a person who for religious reasons does not want the procedure performed. For instance, the starting of an infusion against the will of a rational adult is assault and battery. One must always remember that a rational adult has the right to make his or her decision after pertinent information about the procedure has been provided. If informed consent is not achieved, the patient's desires must be acknowledged and accepted or a tort has occurred. If informed consent is not achieved because of a physical condition or age, the legal statutes of the state must be followed.

So what is the legal standard of care needed by persons who are to receive IV therapy? By definition, the standard of care is that care is given at the level which is expected in the given circumstance in which care is provided. This means that professional care represents what is typical for the person with the knowledge and skill base of the professional. Second, the care must be that given by another health professional with the same education and skill base in the same situation. Finally, the care must be typical of that provided in the geographic area where the care is provided.

Standards of care may be voluntary or may be mandated by governmental departments. The standard of care for IV therapy depends on several factors, including the state medical practices acts, the nursing legislation of the state, the product(s) being infused, and any standards set at the local level such as hospital or agency standards or policies. These local standards should be set forth in policy and procedure manuals, and these should be followed as closely as those from governmental agencies. The person who is providing or monitoring the IV therapy is responsible for the standards of competent care and patient safety.

Patient safety includes the use of infection control recommendations as provided by the Centers for Disease Control and Prevention (CDC) in a publication for prevention of intravascular infections. Other safety standards may be instituted by the local institutions, or the professional standards of certain organizations may enact criteria that must be followed. In all cases, the safety of the patient and risk management must be paramount with IV therapy.

The best of patient care should be expected by the patient and performed by the health care professional. Even in the best of cases, however, mistakes do happen. Just because a mistake has taken place does not mean that malpractice or negligence has happened. Negligence occurs when the person administering IV medications does not act in a reasonable and prudent manner. Malpractice is when the person has been negligent in patient care or the person has deviated from the standards of care that an average health care professional would provide in similar circumstances. Each person is liable for the actions they take, including the physician who initiates the orders for the therapy. Health care professionals should be fully aware of the personal and professional liability that is inherent in providing IV therapy and should adhere to any guidelines that prevent negligence or malpractice. Each professional is responsible and liable for providing the best medical care possible and for taking the care necessary to prevent a variant from the established standard of care.

Just because the initiation of IV therapy is legal, however, does not mean that it is ethical. The health care professional must always ask, "Is this a task that I would do on myself if I could? Would I feel comfortable if I were the patient during this procedure? Are my knowledge and technical bases adequate for patient safety in this situation? Do I know enough about the adverse reactions that I would recognize an adverse reaction?" If the answer is yes in these situations, the health care professional could then decide whether the intravenous therapy could and should be begun and if the knowledge base provides for patient safety. If the answer is no to any of these questions, the health professional should rethink the IV therapy initiation.

RISK MANAGEMENT AND PATIENT CARE WITH INFUSION THERAPY

Risk management is used by health care management to identify, analyze, and then implement strategies to decrease liabilities and to ensure a higher level of patient care. Risk management is a concept that leads to fewer mistakes and takes the mistakes that do happen and provides positive feedback for better patient care. The ideal area of risk management would be that no losses or injuries occur or that exposure to a risk is avoided, but if that is not possible the desire would be to reduce losses and then to prevent that same loss from happening again. Therefore, those who are responsible for risk management look at measures that reduce the possibility of loss, while also looking at ways that patient safety is improved. The tools used should also include measures that prevent further patient injury when a possible injury to a patient has occurred. The health care professional must provide safe treatment, safeguarding any further injury, and must be aware of the indications that need further followup. Instances of the trends of risk should be identified, and interventions for these trends should be found and used to prevent the same risks in the future.

Screening Prior to IV Administration

The responsibilities of the person initiating and monitoring IV therapy include screening the patient prior to the therapy and monitoring the patient before, during, and after the completion of the patient care (Figure 1–1). Before ordering the IV infusion, the physician will perform a baseline screening, including an accurate history, to determine any changes in the physical condition of the patient. This should include not only the patient's health history but a family and social history and a close examination of possible allergies. The person who is beginning the infusion should review this information prior to starting the IV therapy to double-check for any discrepancies in the documented health history and the information gathered during the assessment that might be harmful to the patient.

A clinical screening is equally important and should include a blood pressure determination that may show hypotension resulting from electrolyte changes and fluid loss. Any fluid gain may cause increased blood pressure and increased cardiac output and breathing difficulties. Urine testing to determine the level of hydration, including a routine urinalysis showing the physical properties such as specific gravity, color, and odor, provides the information related to kidney function and the homeostasis of the body. A baseline weight (a total of 1 pound of body weight = 500 mL of fluids) should be obtained and recorded. The person who is dehydrated may have lost weight from the last weight obtained, whereas the person who has edema and needs diuresing will have gained weight. Blood electrolyte studies should also be obtained to determine the needs of electrolyte or fluid replacements.

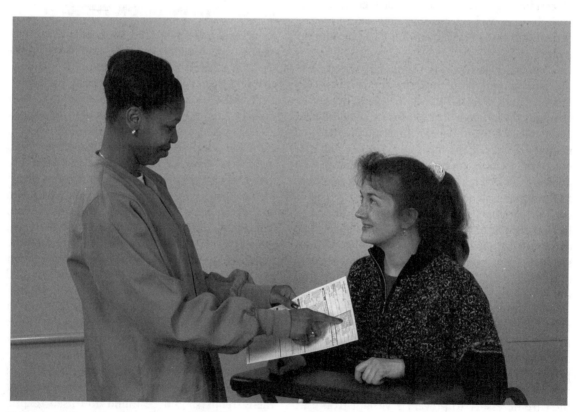

Figure 1-1   Screening the patient prior to IV therapy.

This may include only electrolyte and cell counts or it may be obtained using a complete evaluation of the blood components such as a comprehensive metabolic panel and a complete blood count. In some cases, other testing may be indicated and the physician will order those tests that are necessary.

The patient may also show behavioral changes, such as restlessness and apprehension, when a fluid deficit is evidenced. This may have a gradual onset and not be as apparent as some of the other signs and symptoms of the needs for IV infusion, but this should be evaluated just as the physical symptoms are evaluated. Increased irritability, disorientation, and mental confusion may result from fluid and electrolyte imbalances. Although the screening for these behavioral signs is not legally required, such signs should be documented prior to fluid administration. Belligerence, disorientation, and lethargy should also be documented.

Screening During IV Infusion

The health care professional's responsibilities do not end with the introduction of the IV therapy. Rather, the professional should frequently screen the patient for complications so that early interventions can occur. Complications found may be either local or systemic and include infiltration of the fluids, phlebitis, ecchymosis and hematomas, circulatory system overload, and local infections. The equipment may also be a source of problems, such as malfunctioning electronic infiltration equipment, kinks in the infusion line, or displacement of the infusion devices from the vein; these need attention as quickly as possible.

The health care professional should screen the patient during the treatment by observing and recording results prior to the infusion, during the infusion time, and following the infusion. The patient's observable physical condition and those vital signs appropriate should be taken on a routine basis by a responsible person who is observing the patient during this time for patient safety and good patient care. This provides information at the time of infusion, and it may be the

basis for thwarting legal actions if adverse reactions do occur although the safeguards have been followed. The health care professional must practice within the standard of care for the profession and must remember to follow governmental as well as local and institutional standards of care. That responsibility is important to self and patient and to maintain the level of trust for the profession. With the ability to perform roles of the profession come the responsibilities for proper administration of that professional competency. Those who accept the role for initiating IV therapy must be accountable for responsible patient care.

PATIENT CARE RELATED TO IV THERAPY

Mechanical problems related to the infusion system or trauma to the veins may be the causes of local adverse reactions. Local complications include infiltration of fluids into the surrounding tissues caused by improper placement of the needle, problems with the tubing or solution, trauma to the vein on insertion of the needle, or leaving the tourniquet in place following the connection of the fluids. The patient may be the first person to realize that a problem is occurring because the skin will feel tight and appear stretched and taut. The signs are usually seen close to the insertion site, including slowing or stopping of the fluid infusion, tissue induration, and swelling around the injection site with tissue remaining cool to touch. With the use of infusion devices, the chance of continued infiltration is less likely to occur because an alarm sounds when the fluids infiltrate. If this complication does occur, the infusion site will have to be changed and the affected limb should be elevated and covered with warm compresses or other therapy as ordered by the physician or as directed by the local policies. The health care professional has the responsibility of caring for these complications in a timely manner to prevent further trauma.

Phlebitis, or inflammation of the vein, may occur with infusion therapy, especially if the therapy is given on successive days. Phlebitis is indicated by at least two of the following signs: redness, pain, swelling, and warmth at the site. The inflammation may cause the vein to feel like a cord; this should be found when inspection of the site occurs on a regular basis.

Hematomas and ecchymosis may be found when a tourniquet is placed above the infusion site and is left on after the therapy has started, if the vein is nicked, or if a leaky vein occurs because of frequent use of the same vein. Discoloration of the skin, swelling, and discomfort are the most frequent signs. The health care professional has the responsibility to inspect the infusion site for these complications on a regular, systematic basis. Just because the patient does not complain does not mean that regular care for the site should not take place and that the site is patent.

When IV fluids are infused too rapidly, systemic complications such as cardiac overload and respiratory difficulties may occur. All infusion rates should be responsibly calculated and checked at least twice prior to administration, even if the rate has been calculated by another health care professional. Remember that the person performing the infusion is responsible for his or her actions, including the calculation of the flow rate. Checking infusion speed on a regular basis after the infusion has started is a responsibility that cannot be denied. Each time the patient is checked, the flow rates should also be checked

by the responsible health care professional. Any shortness of breath or swelling should be followed closely with vital signs obtained and the physician notified of the patient's condition on a regular basis if a possible complication has or appears to have occurred.

Intravenous therapy is a common practice in inpatient facilities and is becoming more common in outpatient settings for maintenance, replacement, or restoration therapy. With these duties come responsibilities for good patient care, as well as legal and ethical changes for safety. Constant screening of the patient is essential with IV therapy from the instigation to the time following completion.

REVIEW QUESTIONS

1. What are two of the factors that decide the type of IV fluids that a patient is to receive?
2. What are the goals of IV therapy?
3. Why is the administration of medications by IV route more effective for most medications?
4. Why is the IV route indicated for medications that might be detrimental to tissues?
5. What are the three rationales for IV therapy?
6. Why are cultural and ethnic beliefs so important in the use of IV therapy?
7. What limits the role of the person administering IV therapy?
8. What is meant by standard of care?
9. What is negligence related to medical care and IV therapy? How does this differ from malpractice?
10. Who is liable for the IV therapy?

Chapter 2

Review of Anatomy and Physiology

Chapter Outline

Homeostasis

Circulatory System

Veins Used in IV Therapy

Proximity of Nerves to Veins for IV Therapy

The Lymphatic System

Blood: Its Components and Functions

The Cell

Cellular Regulating Mechanisms

Fluid Balance

Learning Objectives

Upon successful completion of this chapter, the student will be able to:

- Identify and discuss an overview of anatomy and physiology of the entire circulatory system
- Identify and discuss the blood vessels in the upper extremity that are used for therapy
- Discuss homeostasis as it applies to IV therapy

- Identify and discuss the lymphatic system as it pertains to IV therapy
- Discuss peripheral nerves in the arms as they pertain to IV therapy
- Identify and discuss components and functions of blood

Key Terms

aorta—the main trunk arterial vessel (artery) that leaves the left ventricle and carries blood to systemic arteries.

aortic valve—heart valve between left ventricle and aorta.

arterioles—very small arteries at the distal end of the arterial network that carry blood to the capillaries.

artery—blood vessel that carries blood away from the heart that in most cases is oxygenated.

capillaries—minute blood vessels that connect the smallest arterioles to the smallest venules. The walls of capillaries are a single layer of epithelial cells enabling blood and tissue fluid the ability to exchange various substances (gases, fluids, electrolytes, salts, and nutrients).

diffusion—movement of particles or molecules from an area of higher concentration in fluids to one of lower concentration to achieve more equal

distribution of particles/ molecules in the fluid or liquid.

extracellular—outside the cell.

filtration—process in which particles are removed from solution by passing the liquid through a membrane or filter.

homeostasis—state of dynamic balance in the body.

hydrostatic pressure—pressure exerted on a liquid.

inferior vena cava—large vein that collects blood from parts of the body below (inferior to) the heart for return to right atrium.

interstitial—pertaining to space between cells.

interstitial fluids—extracellular fluid in the spaces between body cells providing a substantial portion of liquid environment of the body.

intracellular—within the cell.

intravascular fluids—fluids within the blood vessels.

left atrium—left upper chamber of the heart; receives blood from the pulmonary veins.

left ventricle—left lower chamber of the heart; receives blood from the left atrium.

mitral or bicuspid valve—valve between the left atrium and left ventricle.

osmosis—passage of solvent (fluid) through semipermeable membrane that separates different concentrations of solutions. Movement is from an area where there is a lower concentration of solute into an area where there is an area of higher concentration of solute to equalize the concentration of the two solutions.

plasma—serum, proteins, and chemical substances found in the aqueous portion of blood.

pulmonary circulation—circulation of blood through the lungs for exchange of oxygen and carbon dioxide.

pulmonary (semilunar) valve—valve between the right ventricle and the pulmonary artery.

right atrium—right upper chamber of the heart; receives blood returning to the heart from the inferior and superior vena cava.

right ventricle—right lower chamber of the heart; receives blood from the right atrium.

solute—substance dissolved in a solution.

solvent—solution holding the solute.

superior vena cava—large vein that collects blood from parts of the body above (superior to) the heart for its return to the right atrium.

total parenteral nutrition (TPN)—nutritional support via central access IV therapy to provide glucose, proteins, vitamins, electrolytes, sometimes fats, and so on to maintain the body's growth, development, and tissue repair.

tricuspid valve—valve between the right atrium and right ventricle.

veins—vessels that return blood toward the heart.

venipunctures—puncture of a vein for any purpose; related to IV therapy, puncture of the vein to place an administration device for infusion of IV fluids.

venules—very small veins that carry blood from the capillaries to the veins.

The health care clinician responsible for intravenous (IV) therapy must be cognizant of many aspects of anatomy and physiology, including cell structure; circulatory, lymphatic, and nervous systems; and blood and its components. Reviewing the anatomy of the general cardiovascular system stimulates an awareness of its structures, especially the peripheral vessels, as used with IV therapy. Reassessing the peripheral vascular system and its structures allows the clinician to select an appropriate site for the initiation of IV therapy. Studying the physiology of the circulatory system, including the cardiovascular and peripheral vascular system, helps the clinician to understand the flow of the blood through the body.

Intravenous therapy is not totally dependent on the circulatory system, but includes the relationship with other body systems. Reviewing the involvement of lymph and the lymphatic system helps in understanding the circulation of lymphatic fluid and its relationship to blood in the body. Becoming aware of the nerve structures in the area surrounding the peripheral blood vessels is essential to prevent injury to the nerves at the **venipuncture** site and to reduce patient pain.

Components and properties of blood are also factors in successful IV therapy. Additionally, the clinician should review the role of water, electrolytes, osmolarity, and pH in **homeostasis** of the individual. **Intracellular** fluids (ICF), **extracellular** fluids (ECF), **interstitial fluids**, and the pH of the fluids (such as isotonic fluids, hypotonic fluids, and hypertonic fluids) all are considered for IV therapy and patient safety.

HOMEOSTASIS

Homeostasis is defined as the relative constancy of the internal environment of the human body that is maintained by adaptive responses to promote health and survival. The steady state is maintained through feedback and various sensual mechanisms that provide organs with the needed responses to maintain this internal balance essential for survival. Balance of the body's internal environment includes balancing of body fluids and chemical substances, some of which include electrolytes that are dissolved in body fluids. This dynamic equilibrium between the fluids and electrolytes involves the delicate balance needed to maintain homeostasis and support processes necessary to maintain life. IV therapy is used to maintain homeostasis for those people who for whatever reason have the need for replacement of fluids or electrolytes as well as for medication therapy and blood product replacement.

Body cells are the fundamental functioning unit of the human body. For cells to be able to perform the necessary tasks for maintenance of life, a stable environment, or homeostasis, is necessary. The stability is based on the constant supply of nutrients for the body and the continuous excretion of wastes from metabolism through the urinary, gastrointestinal, or integumentary systems, with some small amounts being lost through respiration. The body fluids lost by removal of body waste must be replaced for homeostasis to be maintained.

Water, accounting for approximately 60% to 75% of total body weight, is the single largest constituent of the body's mass and is essential

to life. Fat cells contain less water, making the percentage of body water dependent on the fat distribution of the person. Age, gender, ethnic origin, and weight also are factors that influence the amount and distribution of body fluids.

Continually moving in the body, water is given different names in various locations, such as intracellular (ICF), extracellular (ECF), plasma, lymph, and interstitial fluid. Homeostasis depends on fluid and electrolyte intake and physiologic factors, disease processes, external factors, and pharmacologic interventions. Electrolytes for homeostasis are dissolved in the blood **plasma**, a body **solvent**, for transport throughout the body. Body fluids are continually exchanged in the intracellular and extracellular sites, such as interstitial spaces and plasma. For a person to remain in fluid homeostasis, that person must maintain an approximately equal intake to output of fluids.

Many of the substances normally found in the body exist in solution, usually aqueous base. The water or fluid is found in different compartments of the body. Intracellular fluid is fluid contained within the cells. Extracellular fluid is found in the spaces between the cells (interstitial space) and in the vascular network as plasma. Fluids have the ability to shift from one area to another, depending on the concentration of electrolytes and proteins in the areas. Fluids will move from an area of lowest concentration of **solutes** to that of the greatest concentration of solutes in a solvent to bring the solution closer to equilibrium of concentration. Examples of consequences of fluid shift include dehydration from vomiting and diarrhea with resulting greater concentration of electrolytes in extracellular spaces. Conversely, fluid retention in the extracellular spaces is treated by restricting sodium and fluid volumes and by drug therapy.

An additional factor in homeostasis or fluid balance is the health status of the person. Dehydration can be caused by extended periods of vomiting or diarrhea, exposure to extreme heat, and reduction of intake of oral fluids. Conditions such as impaired cardiac, renal, or liver function also play an important role in homeostasis. Trauma or surgical procedures may also cause a fluid and/or electrolyte imbalance.

CIRCULATORY SYSTEM

A review of the general circulatory system is vital for patient safety with IV therapy. The anticipation is that this review will provide a recollection of knowledge previously gained.

The heart, located in the thoracic cavity, is situated in the middle of the mediastinal region between the two lungs. It lies behind the sternum and in front of the spinal column. Although the size of the heart varies in each individual, the normal heart, the size of a closed fist, acts as a muscular pump that circulates blood to all tissues of the body.

Route of Blood Flow

Refer to Figures 2–1 and 2–2 for primary routes of the circulation system. The chamber of the heart first receiving carbon dioxide (CO_2)-laden blood from the **superior** and **inferior vena cava** is the right atrium. The blood, moving primarily by

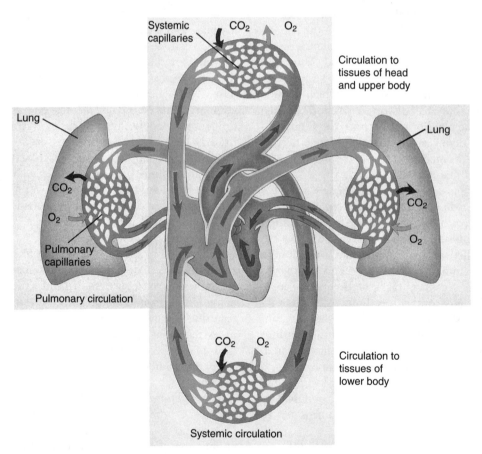

Figure 2-1   Blood flow through the circulatory system. (From Thibodeau GA, Patton KT: *Anthony's textbook of anatomy & physiology,* ed 17, St Louis, 2003, Mosby.)

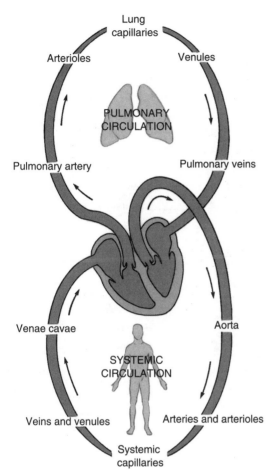

Lung capillaries

Arterioles

Venules

PULMONARY CIRCULATION

Pulmonary artery

Pulmonary veins

Venae cavae

Aorta

SYSTEMIC CIRCULATION

Veins and venules

Arteries and arterioles

Systemic capillaries

Figure 2-2   Scheme of circulatory system. (From Applegate E: *The anatomy and physiology learning system*, ed 3, Philadelphia, 2006, Saunders.) Hint: **Arteries** always carry blood **away** from the heart (the **A**s belong together). **Veins** always carry blood **toward** the heart (This of **TV**).

gravity as the valves open, travels through the **tricuspid valve** into the **right ventricle**. The walls of the atria are thinner than the walls of the ventricles because they do not have to pump the blood into the next area against gravity and to more distant areas of the body as the ventricles do. The right ventricle pumps blood through the **pulmonary (semilunar) valve** into the pulmonary **artery** and then into the lungs, or through **pulmonary circulation**. The blood travels through pulmonary

circulation where gases CO_2 and oxygen (O_2) are exchanged at the cellular level of the alveoli of the lungs. The oxygen-laden blood leaves the pulmonary circulation via the pulmonary **veins** to return to the heart into the **left atrium**. The blood then passes through the **mitral** or **bicuspid valve** into the **left ventricle**. Here, the forceful contraction of the cardiac muscle accelerates the blood through the **aortic valve** into the aorta and into the cardiac and general body or systemic circulation.

The oxygenated blood travels through the systemic circulation to the body via the aorta, which branches to form arteries to the myocardium (or coronary circulation through coronary arteries), brain (through the carotid and cerebral arteries), upper limbs (through brachiocephalic and subclavian arteries), and trunk and lower limbs (via thoracic aorta and femoral arteries) (Figure 2–3 and color insert). As the **aorta** descends into the body, it divides into arteries to supply circulation to the major organ systems and to the peripheral regions of the body. As the arteries branch out, they gradually become smaller and are termed **arterioles**. At the terminal branches of the arterioles, **capillaries** with permeable membranes are formed to allow transfer of nutrients and oxygen into the tissues and absorption of CO_2 and metabolic waste products for return to the heart. The distal end of capillaries become very small veins, called **venules**, and as they progress back to the heart, they turn into progressively larger veins (Figure 2–4 and color insert). The veins terminate in the superior and inferior vena cava to complete the circulatory circuit as they empty deoxygenated blood into the **right atrium** of the heart.

Arteries carry blood away from the heart, and veins return blood to the heart. Systemic arteries are responsible for transporting oxygen-rich blood from the heart to the tissues throughout the body. The only arteries that do not carry oxygen-laden blood are the pulmonary arteries that carry the deoxygenated blood away from the heart to the lungs. This blood, laden with CO_2, will be transported through the pulmonary arteries for exchange of CO_2 and O_2 in the lungs. The pulmonary veins (the only veins that carry

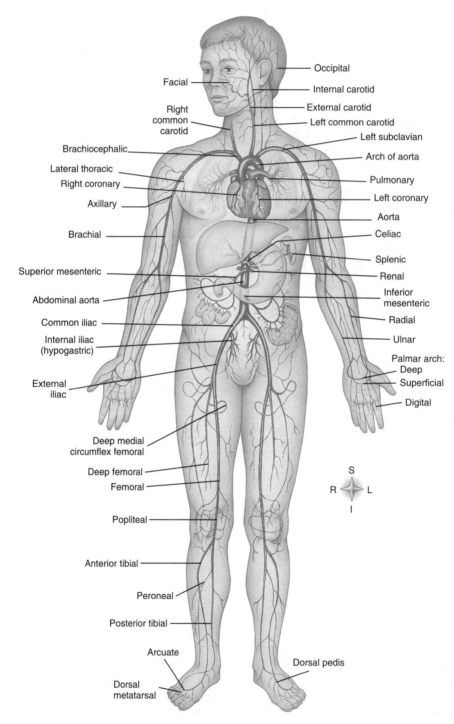

Figure 2-3   Principal arteries of the body. (See color insert.) (From Thibodeau GA, Patton KT: *Anthony's textbook of anatomy & physiology,* ed 17, St Louis, 2003, Mosby.)

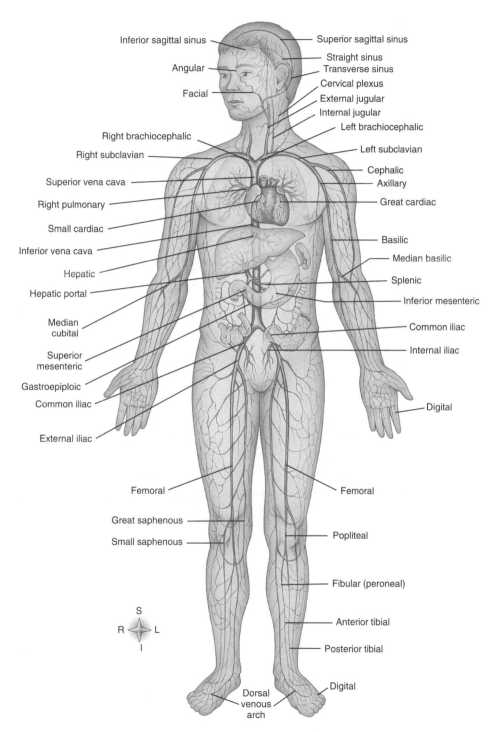

Figure 2-4   Principal veins of the body. (See color insert.) (From Thibodeau GA, Patton KT: *Anthony's textbook of anatomy & physiology,* ed 17, St Louis, 2003, Mosby.)

oxygenated blood) return the oxygen-rich blood back to the left side of the heart for circulation to the body by systemic circulation.

The oxygen-laden blood travels through the arteries to the arterioles and then to the capillaries, where the thin one-celled walls of the capillaries facilitate exchange of gases, nutrients, and solutes into the tissues. The capillaries, residing in tissues, receive waste products of nutrients and CO_2 following metabolism and return these to the blood. The capillaries progress into venules and then veins for the blood to eventually return to the heart via the inferior and superior vena cavae.

Fluid containing solutes leaves the capillaries to surround tissue cells as extracellular fluid.

VEINS USED IN IV THERAPY

IV therapy usually utilizes veins of the hands or arms (and on rare occasions the feet), the subclavian veins on the upper chest wall for catheter placement, and scalp veins for infants and small children (Figure 2–5). There are two classifications for the veins in the arm: superficial and deep. The superficial veins lie near the surface of the skin, whereas the deep veins lie collateral to the arteries in most locations. Veins have valves with cusps, with more in the deeper veins than in the superficial veins. IV therapy usually involves accessing the superficial veins for placement of infusion devices. Deeper veins are usually accessed by a minor surgical procedure, such as placement of percutaneous catheters, which are beyond the scope of this text.

The most distal aspect of the upper extremity venous system in the hands consists of the digital veins that empty into the superficial and deep palmar veins of the hands (Figure 2–5B). These small veins interconnect, forming the palmar venous arches that eventually empty into the cephalic, median antebrachial, and basilic veins.

Veins located in the fingers are identified as digital veins, located along the lateral aspect of the fingers. On occasion, digital veins may be used to initiate IV therapy when a small needle or cannula can be used and when use of the larger veins in the hands and arms is not an immediate option. Small branches of the digital veins eventually join to form the dorsal venous network via the dorsal metacarpal veins between the knuckles on the dorsal aspect or the back of the hand. These are sites that are commonly used to start IVs, especially when a distal site is preferred. These veins are an ideal selection for IV therapy, except for antibiotics, some electrolytes, and chemotherapeutic agents. They are often considered to be the primary choice in patients with hard-to-find veins. If used with geriatric patients, proper support of the site will be required once the infusion is started to prevent movement of the infusion device. The walls of the veins in elderly people are thin and insufficient subcutaneous and muscle tissue are available for support. The veins of the dorsal network eventually flow into the cephalic and basilic veins.

Many of the veins used in IV therapy are superficial lying close to the top of the skin. Some may be a little deeper, but usually veins accessed for the insertion of infusion devices are less than 3 mm deep into the tissue.

Two major superficial veins used for venipuncture and IV therapy are the cephalic and the basilic veins that are located in both the lower and upper arm (Figures 2–5A and 2–7).

The cephalic vein, a large vein that is easily accessed, is situated on the lateral surface of the arm and forearm, lying proximally over the distal lateral aspect of the radius and ascending the forearm on the radial or thumb side of the arm. As the radial vein ascends the lower arm, it joins into the cephalic vein. The cephalic vein eventually goes deep into the upper arm tissue to empty into the subclavian vein.

The basilic vein is located on the ulnar aspect of the forearm, following the ulna and eventually into the upper arm. Similar to the cephalic vein, the large basilic vein ascends up the forearm and then the upper arm, progressing deeper into the tissue to join the brachial vein. This vein is deeper than the cephalic vein and, although easily palpated, it often moves during venipuncture.

Of other veins in the arm, branches of the major veins that may be used include the median

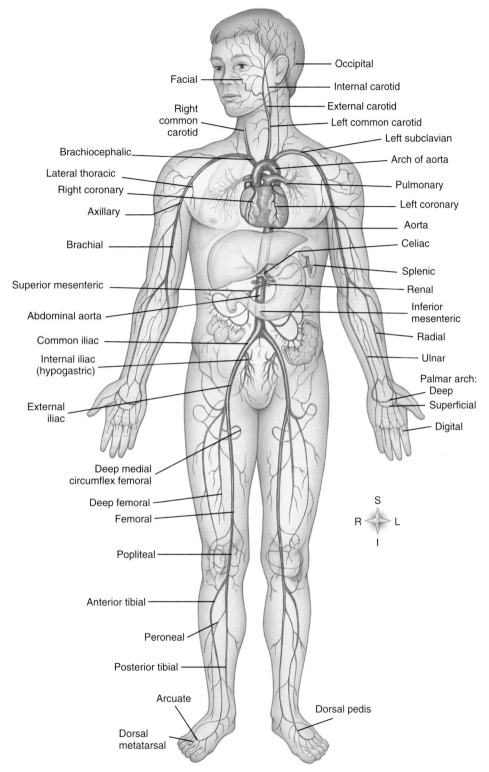

Figure 2-3   Principal arteries of the body. (From Thibodeau GA, Patton KT: *Anthony's textbook of anatomy & physiology,* ed 17, St Louis, 2003, Mosby.)

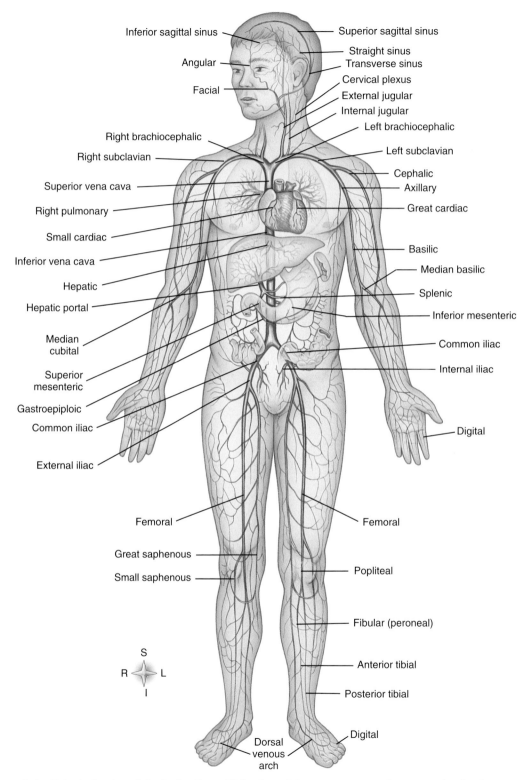

Inferior sagittal sinus

Superior sagittal sinus

Angular

Straight sinus

Transverse sinus

Facial

Cervical plexus

External jugular

Internal jugular

Right brachiocephalic

Left brachiocephalic

Right subclavian

Left subclavian

Superior vena cava

Cephalic

Axillary

Right pulmonary

Great cardiac

Small cardiac

Basilic

Inferior vena cava

Median basilic

Hepatic

Splenic

Hepatic portal

Inferior mesenteric

Median
cubital

Common iliac

Superior
mesenteric

Internal iliac

Gastroepiploic

Common iliac

Digital

External iliac

Femoral

Femoral

Great saphenous

Small saphenous

Popliteal

Fibular (peroneal)

Anterior tibial

Posterior tibial

Digital

Dorsal
venous
arch

S

R ◇ L

I

Figure 2-4   Principal veins of the body. (From Thibodeau GA, Patton KT: *Anthony's textbook of anatomy & physiology,* ed 17, St Louis, 2003, Mosby.)

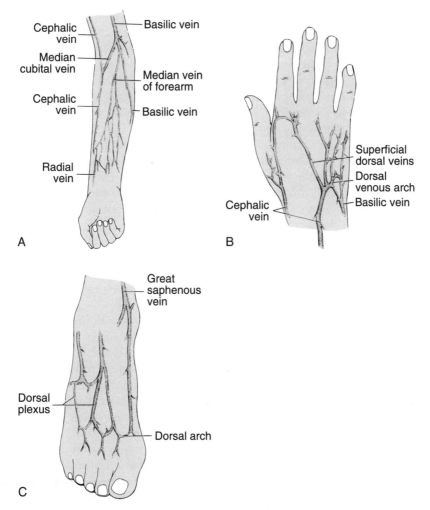

Figure 2-5   Common IV sites. **A,** Inner arm. **B,** Dorsal surface of hand. **C,** Dorsal surface of foot. (From Perry AG, Potter PA: *Basic nursing: Essentials for practice,* ed 5, St Louis, 2003, Mosby.)

cubital and the median vein. Refer to Figure 2–4 (or color insert) for an overview of superficial veins of the left upper limb. These veins form branches identified as the median cubital vein and the median vein. Another vein that is accessed for venipuncture is the median cubital vein, which is palpated and found on the anterior surface of the inner aspect of the elbow. The median cubital vein ascends the arm from the cephalic vein and crosses in front of the brachial artery in the antecubital space to connect with the basilic vein. It also divides above the antecubital fossa, forming the deep brachial vein. The median cubital vein is close to the skin and lying across the antecubital fossa. Because of its larger size and because it is well-anchored, the median cubital vein frequently is used for venipuncture by phlebotomists and is a good site for IV therapy.

The median vein, also referred to as the median antebrachial vein, arises from the veins of the palmer area of the hand and ascends the ulnar side of the front of the lower arm. This vein terminates into the basilic vein or the median cubital vein. Occasionally, it will divide into two branches, one branch joining the basilic vein and the other branch joining the cephalic vein below the elbow. This vein is found in an area with many nerve endings and thus should be avoided for IV therapy if possible.

Veins in the feet may be used when venous access in the arms and hands is not an option, such as a case of amputation (Figure 2–5C). The digital veins in the feet flow from the toes and form the dorsal venous arch, much like the digital veins form the arch in the hands. The dorsal veins of the foot arise from these veins and progress to form the anterior tibial vein, the great and small saphenous veins, and the posterior tibial vein.

Other medical situations may require an atypical use of veins for IV therapy. Scalp veins are used in infants and very young children. The subclavian vein, located in the shoulder underlying the clavicle, is usually a surgical option for placing central venous catheters and is used for those patients with veins that are difficult to access or for long-term therapy to prevent repeated venipunctures. These catheters or continuous access ports are placed for continuous or intermittent infusions or for administration of high volume or viscous products, such as **total parenteral nutrition (TPN)**. Chemotherapy, antimicrobials, and analgesics may be administered via this route. Because specialized training is recommended before attempting subclavian approaches, discussion of this option is beyond the scope of this text.

Veins often are located running parallel to arteries. Care must be taken to not confuse one with the other. The distinction between an artery and a vein can be identified by the following hints. These comparisons include the color of blood in each: dark red in veins and bright red in arteries. Venous blood will provide a slow, steady blood return in the infusion administration device, whereas arterial blood generates a

rapid, pulsating blood return. Veins have valves at the point of branching and at other locations at approximately every three inches in the vein, whereas arteries have no valves. Valves or cusps help the vascular network to resist the forces of gravity on the flow of blood to prevent backward flow on the return of blood to the heart. Veins used for IV therapy are usually in a superficial location, whereas arteries are usually in a deeper location and surrounded by muscle. Multiple veins absorb blood from an area of tissue, whereas a single artery usually provides blood supply to an area of tissue. Other important distinctions between veins and arteries include the following:

- Arteries are thick-walled and veins have thinner walls.
- Each have three tissue levels (these are 25% of the total diameter of arteries and only 10% of veins).
- Veins have the ability to distend to a greater degree, allowing for storage of large amounts of blood.
- About 25% of the body's blood is found in veins.

When considering venous anatomy before initiating the IV, certain aspects should be considered. Unless it is an emergent situation where access to a large vein is required to administer blood or blood products by rapid infusion, distal veins of the hands or lower arms should be considered as the first option. This is the optimum consideration because it preserves the integrity of the proximal veins for access at a later time for additional IV therapy. Assessment of the anticipated site should include an unused vein that is reasonably straight. A successful venipuncture depends on careful vein selection and assessment for a vein that is easily palpated and is reasonably straight.

Structure of Blood Vessels

Veins and arteries are composed of three concentric layers (Figure 2–6). The multiple layers of tissue provide the vessels with strength and permit changes in the diameter of the vessels as required with vascular pressure and volume changes. The inner layer of blood vessel walls is the tunica

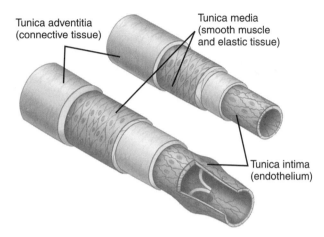

Tunica adventitia
(connective tissue)

Tunica media
(smooth muscle
and elastic tissue)

Tunica intima
(endothelium)

Figure 2-6   Structure of blood vessels. (**A**) Vein, (**B**) Artery. (From Thibodeau GA, Patton KT: *Anthony's textbook of anatomy & physiology,* ed 17, St Louis, 2003, Mosby.)

intima; the middle layer is the tunica media; and the external or outermost layer is the tunica adventitia (externa). In veins, the tunica intima usually is smooth with no elastic membrane present. Valves in the veins are actually folds of this layer (tunica intima) projecting from the vessel wall and pointing in the direction of blood flow toward the heart. The middle layer or tunica media of veins is thin and contains smooth-muscle and collagen fibers that are inundated to produce vasodilation and vasoconstriction. The outer layer or tunica externa of veins consists of collagen, elastic, and smooth-muscle fibers that surround and support the vessel. Veins have a tendency to collapse when not under pressure or distended by blood; therefore, some pressure is always present on the walls of the veins to prevent collapse. Diastolic blood pressure is responsible for the distention and, therefore, it always is above zero.

Blood pressure in veins normally is lower than in arteries and does not have sufficient pressure to oppose the force of gravity. The valves located in the tunica intima permit the blood to flow in one direction, toward the heart, and prevent any backward flow into the capillaries. The valves keep the blood "compartmentalized" into these areas between the veins, thus dividing the amount and weight of the blood throughout the vessels,

limiting distention. Movement of the muscles surrounding the veins causes the walls to compress and the blood to be moved to the next valvular area. A slight distension may be noted in the wall of the vein where the valve is located.

PROXIMITY OF NERVES TO VEINS FOR IV THERAPY

Knowledge of the relationship between vein and nerve locations in the upper limbs is essential for the practitioner initiating an IV. Care must be taken to prevent damage to a nerve during the venipuncture process. Additionally, considering the close proximity of a nerve to the vein of the intended site may prevent unnecessary pain for the patient. Refer to Figure 2–7 for an overview of proximity of veins and the major veins of the upper limb.

Many facilities now use a mini-ultrasound device at the bedside to locate veins before attempting to start an infusion. It is usually handheld and portable for convenience of the operator. These devices use ultrasound technology to locate and identify vascular structures and to assist the clinician in differentiating between vessels and nerves.

The clinician should be aware that problems may evolve as a result of insult to the peripheral nerves. Trauma to peripheral nerves usually causes

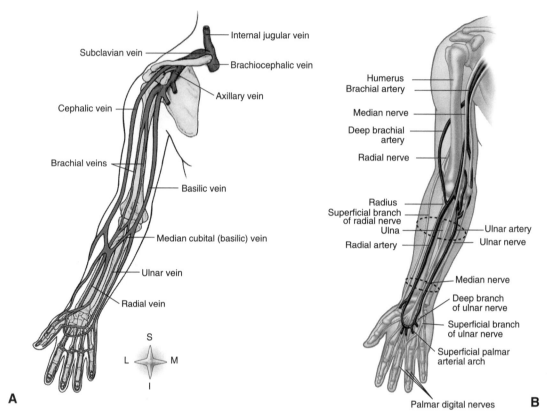

Figure 2-7   Proximity of the major veins and nerves of the upper extremity. (**A** from Thibodeau GA, Patton KT: *Anthony's textbook of anatomy & physiology,* ed 17, St Louis, 2003, Mosby; **B** from Dorland's Illustrated Medical Dictionary, ed 30, Philadelphia, 2003, Saunders.)

noticeable pain, as may edema in the area. Trauma or edema may cause a loss of function of the muscles supplied by the nerve that has suffered an insult.

Major nerves in the arms include the radial nerve on the lateral aspect of the arm that travels along the radius in the lower arm, terminating in the lateral aspect of the thumb. The median nerve travels between the radius and the ulna in the middle of the anterior region of the arm, past the distal aspect of each bone and terminating in the medial aspect of the thumb, the second and third digits, and the lateral aspect of the fourth digit. The ulnar nerve lies on the medial aspect of the arm and travels down the arm alongside the ulna, past the distal aspect of the ulna and terminating in the medial aspect of the fourth digit and

the entire fifth digit. Knowing the location of these peripheral nerves and their proximity to vessels will be helpful in avoiding damage.

THE LYMPHATIC SYSTEM

The lymphatic system also plays a role in the circulation of body fluids. Lymph, a fluid similar to plasma, contains a lower concentration of suspended proteins in its aqueous base. Much of the tissue fluid filtrate is absorbed by blood vessel capillaries through the process of osmosis. However, the remaining fluid is filtered from the interstitial spaces, is absorbed into the lymph for transport back to the circulatory system through the lymphatic vessels to become part of the circulating blood.

This thin, watery fluid develops in body organs and tissues and is filtered by lymph nodes as it circulates through the lymphatic system. The lymphatic vessels usually flow close to the blood vessels and join the circulatory veins at the junction of the internal jugular and subclavian veins. This vast network of lymphatic capillaries and vessels helps to maintain the internal fluid environment of the body, thus playing an important role in homeostasis.

Similar to veins, the lymphatic vessels have valves to prevent the backward flow of the lymph and to keep it progressing through the lymphatic system.

BLOOD: ITS COMPONENTS AND FUNCTIONS

The state of well-being, optimum health, and even survival of the human body is dependent on homeostasis, maintained by nutrients and fluids in the blood. Therefore, discussion of the circulatory system would not be complete without consideration of blood, its components, characteristics, functions, and role in homeostasis.

Blood is composed of two major components: formed elements or solids and liquid or plasma. The formed elements consist of red blood cells (erythrocytes), white blood cells (leukocytes), and platelets (thrombocytes) and the liquid portion consists of about 90% water and organic and inorganic solutes that are dissolved in the liquid with its solvent abilities. The solutes are in a constant state of change as a result of cellular activity by the body functions. An understanding of the importance of homeostasis provides reasoning for the maintenance of fluid and electrolyte balance by the dispersion of needed solvents and solutes in the blood for maintenance of the health of the person.

Blood, as a connective tissue, is composed of solids in the form of cells and cell fragments and of plasma, the liquid portion. Blood provides the transport medium necessary to support life through nutrition and excretion of waste products and is involved in regulation activities and in protection of the body to maintain homeostasis.

It is difficult to categorize and distinguish a separation of these activities because they overlap.

The transportation function includes carrying nutrients and oxygen to the cells, hormones to target tissues, carbon dioxide to the lungs, and other waste products of cellular metabolism to the kidneys for elimination. Involved in regulation of body functions, the blood maintains body temperature, fluid and electrolyte balance, and balance of the pH of the body. As a source of protection for the body, blood plays an active role in the clotting process and specific blood cells, called phagocytes, target invading microorganisms to prevent infection and disease. Other cells in the blood plasma, antibodies, also help to fend off disease as they react to invading microorganisms.

A major function of red blood cells (erythrocytes) is transportation of oxygen from the lungs to the systemic cells, as hemoglobin in the erythrocytes combines with the oxygen for transport to the cells in the body. These cells also pick up some carbon dioxide in the systemic circulation and carry it back to the lungs, where it is released to be exhaled from the body.

Leukocytes rely on the plasma of the blood for transport to body tissue where they perform their assigned duties. Some leukocytes are phagocytic in action, some stimulate the production of antibodies, others are responsible for the secretion of histamine and heparin, and others function to neutralize heparin. Leukocytes have the ability to travel through capillary walls into tissue spaces, where they work to provide a defense against invading microorganisms or they may be involved in the promotion or inhibition of the inflammatory process.

Platelets (thrombocytes) are small fragments of large cells, megakaryocytes. Platelets have the ability and tendency to become sticky and clump together (aggregate), forming platelet plugs. These cells have the ability to plug breaks and tears in blood vessels and to initiate the formation of blood clots.

Many solutes are dissolved in plasma. Plasma proteins include albumins, globulins, and fibrinogen (Figure 2–8). Nitrogenous molecules include amino acids, urea, and uric acids. Other dissolved solutes are nutrients, electrolytes, antibodies,

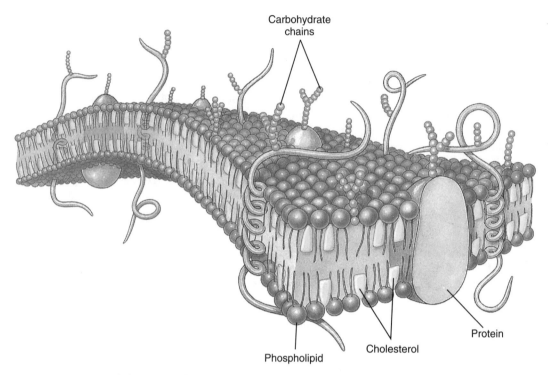

Figure 2-8 Structure of plasma membrane. (From Thibodeau GA, Patton KT: *Structure and function of the body,* ed 12, St Louis, 2004, Mosby.)

carbon dioxide, oxygen, and hormones. Globulins transport lipids and fat-soluble materials. Gamma globulins play a role in immunity. Fibrinogen is part of the blood-clotting process.

Albumin has an important role in the maintenance of fluid balance between blood and interstitial fluid. As a carrier molecule, albumin is necessary to maintain blood volume, blood pressure, and osmotic pressure in the capillaries. This prevents loss of plasma from the capillaries while maintaining the pressure needed to keep capillaries patent. When osmotic pressure of the blood decreases, fluid will move from the blood into the interstitial spaces, creating edema. A decrease in blood volume occurs, to be followed by falling blood pressure. Conversely, if blood osmotic pressure increases, fluid will move from the interstitial space into the blood to increase blood volume. An increase in blood

volume occurs, to be followed by rising blood pressure and decreasing amounts of water available to the cells. Thus, albumin may be used in emergency situations to maintain blood volume and blood pressure.

Electrolytes play a significant role in homeostasis. Sodium, potassium, calcium bicarbonate, and phosphate are common electrolytes or solutes found in plasma. The electrolytes are organic ions that help to maintain membrane potentials and regulation of the pH of body fluids.

The average adult female has approximately 4 to 5 L of blood, and the adult male has 5 to 6 L. Under normal circumstances, the total volume of blood is circulated through the system every minute. Blood is 4 to 5 times more viscous than water and is slightly alkaline. Under normal circumstances, the pH of blood is 7.35 to 7.45.

THE CELL

The cell, the primary functional unit in the human body, has structural, physiologic, and developmental functions. Cells may have different characteristics according to the purpose they serve in the body including breathing, digesting, excreting, transporting, supporting, and reproducing. Essentially, they are all similar in structure; however, each type tends to look different according to their specific function (Figure 2–9).

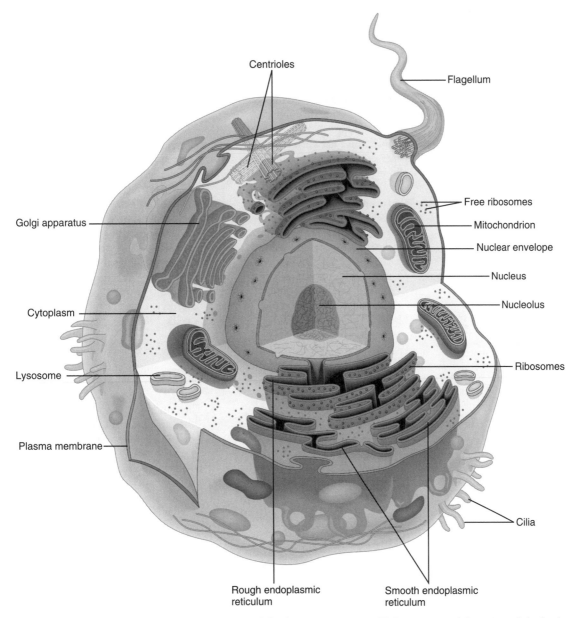

Figure 2-9   Characteristics of the cell. (From Thibodeau GA, Patton KT: *Structure and function of the body,* ed 12, St Louis, 2004, Mosby.)

Table 2-1 STRUCTURE AND FUNCTION OF SOME MAJOR CELL PARTS

Cell Part	Structure	Function(s)
Plasma membrane	Phospholipid bilayer studded with proteins	Serves as the boundary of the cell; protein and carbohydrate molecules on the outer surface of plasma membrane perform various functions; for example, they serve as markers that identify cells of each individual or as receptor molecules for certain hormones
Ribosomes	Tiny particles each made up of rRNA (ribosomal ribonucleic acid) subunits	Synthesize proteins; a cell's "protein factories"
Endoplasmic reticulum (ER)	Membranous network of interconnected canals and sacs, some with ribosomes attached (rough ER) and some without attachments (smooth ER)	Rough ER receives and transports reticulum (ER) synthesized proteins (from ribosomes); smooth ER synthesizes lipids and (rough ER) and some certain carbohydrates
Golgi apparatus	Stack of flattened, membranous sacs	Chemically processes then packages substances from the ER
Mitochondria	Membranous capsule containing a large, folded membrane encrusted with enzymes	ATP (adenosine triphosphate) synthesis; a cell's "powerhouses"
Lysosomes	"Bubble" of enzymes encased by membrane	A cell's "digestive system"
Centrioles	Pair of hollow cylinders, each made up of tiny tubules	Function in cell reproduction
Cilia	Short, hairlike extensions on a surface of some cells	Move substances over surface of the cell
Flagella	Single and much longer projection of some cells	The only example in humans is the "tail" of a sperm cell, propelling the sperm through fluids
Nucleus	Double-membraned, spherical envelope containing DNA strands	Dictates protein synthesis, thereby playing an essential role in other cell activities, namely active transport, metabolism, growth, and heredity
Nucleoli	Dense region of the nucleus	Play an essential role in the formation of ribosomes

Modified from Thibodeau GA, Patton KT: *Structure and function of the body,* ed 12, St Louis, 2004, Mosby.

In the human body, some cells may be in remote areas and are therefore dependent on circulating fluids to carry oxygen and nourishment to them and to transport waste materials of metabolism away. The various systems or groups of cells of the body carry on the biological activities of the body as a complete organism.

Each cell is encompassed in a very thin and delicate cell membrane or wall. This cell wall encompasses cytoplasm containing minute organelles or granules of various sizes. Inside the cell is the nucleus, which controls metabolism, provides storage, and processes genetic information. The cells are contained or float in extracellular fluid. The cell structure is dependent on and specific to the function of the cell. (Table 2–1 indicates the components found in cell structure and the function of the structures.)

CELLULAR REGULATING MECHANISMS

Homeostasis of fluids or body water balance depends on intake of fluid sources and elimination of waste from the body. Intake of water includes water contained in food, water consumed in liquid form, and water resulting from oxidation. Water is excreted from the body through the skin, through the lungs during respiration, and in feces and urine. The average individual takes in approximately 2500 mL of fluid in a 24-hour period and excretes approximately the same amount. For cells to maintain the balance of intake and excretion, the fluids must move into and out of cells by various processes.

It is through the semipermeable membranes of the cell walls that fluids move in and out of the cells. The fluid contained within the cell walls is referred to as intracellular fluid (ICF) and that whichis outside the cell wall is extracellular fluid (ECF). The ECF is in the interstitial space. These fluids move across the cell walls by **diffusion, osmosis,** and **filtration** (Table 2–2).

Diffusion

During the process of diffusion, particles or molecules move from an area of higher concentration of fluids to an area of lower concentration until equal distribution in the fluid is achieved (Figure 2–10). At the capillary level, gases (O_2 and CO_2) are exchanged by diffusion.

Osmosis

The process of osmosis is the passage or diffusion of solvent through a selectively semipermeable

Table 2-2 PASSIVE TRANSPORT PROCESSES

Process	Description	Examples
Diffusion	Movement of particles through a membrane from an area of high concentration to an area of low concentration—that is, down the concentration gradient	Movement of carbon dioxide out of all cells; movement of sodium ions into nerve cells as they conduct an impulse
Osmosis	Diffusion of water through a selectively permeable membrane in the presence of at least one impermeable solute	Diffusion of water molecules into and out of cells to correct imbalances in water concentration
Filtration	Movement of water and small solute particles, but not larger particles, through a filtration membrane; movement occurs from area of high pressure to area of low pressure	In the kidney, movement of water and small solutes from blood vessels but lack of movement by blood proteins and blood cells; begins the formation of urine

Modified from Thibodeau GA, Patton KT: *Structure and function of the body,* ed 12, St Louis, 2004, Mosby.

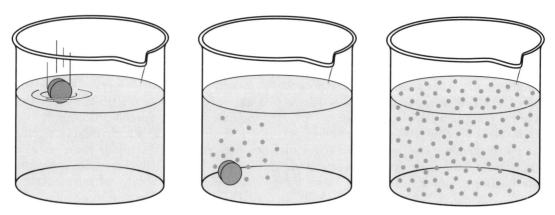

Figure 2-10   Simple diffusion. (From Applegate E: *The anatomy and physiology learning system,* ed 2, Philadelphia, 2000, Saunders.)

membrane that separates different concentrations. Movement is from an area of higher concentration of water molecules into an area of lower concentration of water molecules (Figure 2–11).

Osmosis, responsible for approximately 50% of the body's homeostasis, is complete when equilibrium is reached and the solution on both sides of the membrane has the same concentration of solutes, as every fluid in the body seeks to be isotonic. An example is arterial blood that is hypertonic in its concentration of oxygen and hypotonic in its concentration of waste products.

Filtration

Filtration involves the movement of solution through a membrane or filter to remove particles from the solution, involving the use of mechanical pressure. The water and dissolved materials are forced through a membrane in an area of higher pressure to an area of lower pressure.

In blood, filtration occurs as blood flows through capillaries that have one-cell permeable walls. Capillary blood pressure is higher than tissue pressure, so that force pushes plasma and nutrients out of the capillaries into tissue fluids. As previously stated, albumin at the venous end of the capillaries pulls tissue fluids back into the capillaries, bringing in the waste products for excretion.

FLUID BALANCE

There are three states of concentration of solutes in body fluids: isotonic fluids, hypotonic fluids, and hypertonic fluids. Isotonic fluids are when the solutes in the fluids constitute a neutral state or the normal state of fluids in the body at 0.9% saline.

During the process of diffusion, molecules move from an area of high concentration to an area of lower concentration to form isotonic solutions. This action or movement continues until the molecules are evenly distributed and equilibrium of the fluids exists. Diffusion may occur across a membrane as long as the membrane is permeable. Diffusion of substances through extracellular and intracellular fluids of the body takes place through the process of diffusion.

Hypotonic is when the concentration of solutes is lower than normal/neutral body fluids. Hypertonic is the state that occurs when the solutes are in greater concentration than body fluids.

An example is the concentration of saline in relationship to body fluids/blood. Saline concentration of body fluids is normal at 0.9% of sodium and chloride electrolytes. IV solution identified as normal saline is the isotonic or neutral solution, and it usually is used for fluid and electrolyte replacement. When hypotonic or hypertonic fluid

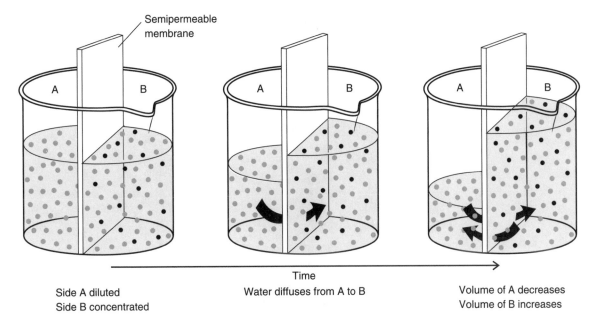

Figure 2-11   Osmosis. (From Applegate E: *The anatomy and physiology learning system*, ed 2, Philadelphia, 2000, Saunders.)

concentrates are used for replacement, it is possible that blood cells will be destroyed because the cells either shrivel up as a result of loss of water (crenate) or the opposite—when they take up water and swell and the cell membrane ruptures (lysis) (Figure 2–12). When the rupture occurs in a red blood cell it is termed hemolysis.

Isotonic fluids have a similar osmolarity as serum; thus, no fluid movement occurs. Isotonic fluids remain in the **intravascular** compartment with a resulting expansion of the compartment, or allow fluids to remain in ECF spaces and expand these also. There is no shift of fluids between compartments. This concept is used in treating patients who need to expand the extravascular compartments. Using caution is necessary to prevent fluid overload. Patients with congestive heart failure and hypertension are at risk of fluid overload and its consequences. Examples of isotonic IV solutions include

lactated Ringer's solution or 0.9% saline in water (normal saline).

Hypotonic IV solutions have less osmolarity than serum, thus subsequently diluting the serum and decreasing its osmolarity (Figure 2–13). Water moves from the vascular compartment into the interstitial fluid compartment. Interstitial fluid is diluted and the concentration of active particles in the fluids (osmolarity) decreases, drawing water into the adjacent cells. This concept is used to treat patients whose cells are dehydrated or in hyperglycemic situations including diabetic ketoacidosis when high serum glucose levels have drawn fluid out of the cells moving the fluid out of interstitial spaces and into vascular and interstitial compartments. This type of therapy carries risks with the sudden fluid shift from the intravascular space into the cells. The resulting consequences can be cardiovascular collapse or increased intracranial pressure in certain patients.

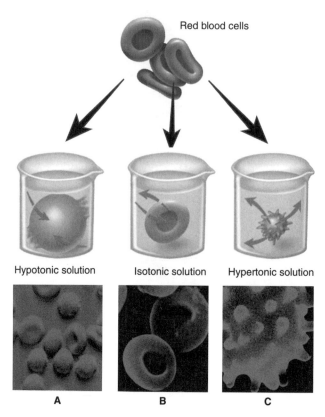

Figure 2-12 Effects of toxicity on cells. (From Thibodeau GA, Patton KT: *Anthony's textbook of anatomy & physiology,* ed 17, St Louis, 2003, Mosby.)

Examples of hypotonic IV solutions include 0.45% sodium chloride and 2.5% dextrose solutions.

Hypertonic solutions have higher osmolarity levels than serum, resulting in fluids and electrolytes being pulled from the intracellular and

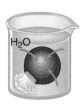 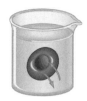

Figure 2-13 Tonicity. (From Thibodeau GA, Patton KT: *Structure and function of the body,* ed 12, St Louis, 2004, Mosby.)

interstitial compartments into the intravascular compartment. These fluids can help stabilize blood pressure with resulting increased urine output and reduced edema. Hypertonic solution therapy is rarely used in the prehospital setting because caution must be taken because they are more dangerous to use. Some hypertonic IV solutions are D5% 0.45% NaCl, D5% LR, D5% NS, blood products, and albumin. See Table 2–3 for toxicity of common intravenous fluids.

The clinician responsible for IV therapy has a responsibility to be as knowledgeable as possible about the anatomy and physiology of the circulatory system and homeostasis when administering IV fluids. The role of water in the body's function requires an in-depth understanding. Diffusion, osmosis, filtration, and tonicity all play a role in homeostasis. IV therapy is therapeutic

Table 2-3   COMMON SOLUTIONS USED FOR INTRAVENOUS ADMINISTRATION

Solution	Terms for Isotonic Solutions	Terms for Hypotonic Solutions	Terms for Hypertonic Solutions
Saline	0.9% sodium chloride Normal saline (NS) 0.9% NaCl/0.9% NS	0.45% sodium chloride ½ Strength NS/½ NaCl 0.45% NS/0.45% NaCl	3%–5% sodium chloride
Dextrose in NaCl	5% Dextrose in NS D-5-NS	5% Dextrose in ½ NaCl D-5-½ NaCl D-5-0.45% NS	
Dextrose in water	5% Dextrose in water D-5-W	2.5% Dextrose in water D-2.5-W	10% Dextrose in water D-10-W
Lactated Ringer's solution	Lactated Ringer's solution LR		5% Dextrose in lactated Ringer's solution D-5-LR

From Fulcher EM, Soto CD, Fulcher RM: Pharmacology: principles and applications, Philadelphia, 2003, Saunders.

in nature and the patient's state of health should not be compromised.

REVIEW QUESTIONS

1. Discuss homeostasis as related to IV therapy.
2. Describe the circulation of blood in general circulation.
3. Describe the function of arteries and veins.
4. Explain the role of capillaries.
5. Discuss the structure of veins.
6. What is the function of valves in the veins?
7. List the functions of blood.
8. Define and discuss osmosis.
9. Compare the three states of solutes in solutions and explain the effects of hypertonic solution and hypotonic solution on blood cells.
10. Compare intracellular and extracellular fluids.

3
Review of Asepsis

Chapter Outline

Proper Hygiene/Disinfection

Types of Pathogens

Chain of Infection

Medical Asepsis

Surgical Asepsis

Necessity of Sterile Technique with IV Fluids

Using Medical Asepsis to Prepare for IV Therapy

Universal Precautions

OSHA Bloodborne Pathogens Standards

Summary of the Need for Asepsis

Learning Objectives

Upon successful completion of this chapter, the student will be able to:

- Explain the importance of quality hand hygiene.
- Explain the difference between medical aseptic technique and sterile technique.
- Discuss the importance of maintaining sterile technique in the administration of IV fluids.

- List and discuss Universal Precautions related to IV therapy.
- List and discuss OSHA regulations related to IV therapy.

Key Terms

bloodborne pathogens—microorganisms capable of causing disease in humans and transmitted in human blood.

contaminated—no longer sterile, soiled, unclean.

exposure incident—occurrence when the clinician is exposed to a potent

bloodborne pathogen from body fluids.

medical asepsis—clean techniques to decrease pathogens to reduce the incidence of cross-contamination; also known as the clean technique.

nosocomial infection—infection acquired in health care setting.

occupational exposure—being exposed to harmful microorganisms or other harmful factors through employment.

surgical asepsis—using sterile technique; to use methods to kill all microorganisms in a given situation.

I nfection control is a major factor in patient safety with intravenous (IV) therapy. Hand washing/hand hygiene, medical asepsis, and sterile technique all play a part in infection control. Compliance with Occupational Safety and Health Administration (OSHA) guidelines and Universal Precautions also contribute to initiating and maintaining infection control. Other factors that may affect the incidence of infection in a patient include natural defenses against infection such as an intact skin, a functional immune system, and the person's general state of good health (or homeostasis). Additionally, the type of microorganism and its state of mutation for antibiotic resistance are involved in the progression or arresting of an infection.

PROPER HYGIENE/DISINFECTION

The incidence of infection can be reduced by the use of both aseptic and sterile techniques. The health care professional who has the responsibility for initiating or caring for an IV must practice both techniques and be cognizant of both of these techniques at all times to maintain patient safety.

Microorganisms can be pathogenic or nonpathogenic with disease-producing organisms being identified as pathogens. **Medical asepsis** refers to an area or object that is free from pathogens. It is possible for nonpathogens to be present on a medical aseptic or clean surface. Proper disinfection of an area and hand washing are key elements in medical aseptic technique.

Hand Hygiene

Historically, cleansing of the hands has been referred to in the traditional term of hand washing. With the advent of antimicrobial hand sanitizing agents, the term hand hygiene has become the term of choice. A thorough washing of hands with soap and warm water at the beginning of the workday and several times throughout the day is still recommended. However, it is acceptable to use the waterless, alcohol-based antimicrobial scrub/wash between hand washing when clean hands are essential. The prevention of nosocomial infection is the goal of excellent health care, and hand hygiene plays an important role in that goal. It is good practice to review proper hand washing techniques on a regular basis and to practice them daily, according to aseptic technique. Basic infection control practices must be followed at all times by all personnel for infection control.

Other factors to be considered in appropriate hand hygiene include the length of the nails and the use of nail polish. Nails should be smooth and should not extend over the end of the fingertip. Long nails may puncture the tips of latex or other protective gloves. Acrylic or artificial nails should not be on the fingertips because these additions may harbor fungus and other microorganisms, resulting in infections. If polish is used, it should be clear so the underside of the nail tips can be seen and examined for the presence of dirt or foreign matter. Nail polish should be free of any chips. Rings should not be worn because they also may harbor pathogens under the band or in mountings for stones.

Cleansing Agents

Altering the conditions that allow pathogens to live, multiply, and spread eliminates infectious pathogens. This can be accomplished by the use of disinfectants and antiseptic preparations.

Disinfectants are chemical preparations used to kill or eliminate pathogens from objects. They do not have the capability of killing bacterial spores. Often referred to as germicides or bactericides, these products kill living and active microorganisms. As a result of the chemical strength, disinfectants are usually not used on skin or mucous membranes. Their intended action is to kill microorganisms on inanimate objects such as equipment, environmental surroundings, and supplies. Examples of disinfectants are full-strength household bleach, phenol, and formaldehyde. When using these solutions, the health care provider should take protective skin precautions such as wearing gloves and using splash protection equipment.

Antiseptics tend to inhibit the growth and reproduction of microorganisms; however, they do not completely kill microorganisms. Antiseptics interfere with cellular metabolism, thus preventing survival and replication. These products can be applied to skin and mucous membranes. Additionally, they may be used as cleansing agents. Examples of antiseptics are 70% isopropyl alcohol, iodine preparations, and chlorhexidine gluconate. Caution must be exercised when using iodine preparations on patients because many individuals are allergic to iodine. Prior to use, the patient must be questioned about the incidence of any reaction, local or systemic, to iodine and evaluate these reactions, if applicable. The clinician must constantly observe the site where the iodine preparation was applied for any local reaction, such as itching or a rash at the site. Additionally, they must be aware of any signs of possible systemic reaction, such as hives, difficulty breathing, or other signs of allergic reaction.

TYPES OF PATHOGENS

The skin harbors numerous pathogens and non-pathogens. The staphylococcal bacteria *Staphylococcus aureus* are frequently found on the skin and are often the cause of infections that enter the body through the catheter lumen or the outside of the catheter. This pathogen is found on many surfaces of the clinical environment and on pieces of equipment. Other pathogens or common microorganisms responsible for nosocomial infections are *Pseudomonas aeruginosa*, *Escherichia coli, enterococci,* and staphylococci with *Staphylococcus epidermis* responsible for many infections. Although these microorganisms reside on the skin the majority of the time, they usually do not become pathogens until they enter the bloodstream or a body cavity. Another frequently found and considered almost-normal flora found on body surfaces is a fungus, *Candida albicans.* Subsequent fungal infection can be the result of introduction of the pathogen by **contaminated** fluids, equipment,

or cross-infection or from colonized hands of clinicians.

A case in point deals with a neonate who was respiratory compromised and in a neonatal intensive care unit (NICU) receiving IV fluids. The infant developed a **nosocomial infection** in the second week of life and subsequently died. Cultures obtained during the illness identified *Candida albicans* as the causative agent. Among the items used in his care, the IV tubing tested positive for *Candida albicans* as did one of the care provider's hands. Proper hand sanitizing technique and proper frequency may have prevented the nosocomial infection and the infant's demise.

The presence of normal body flora on the skin is always a factor in the possibility of infection during IV therapy, because the normal flora may be injected under the skin as it is punctured by the needle (Figure 3–1). Proper cleansing of the skin prior to the initiation of the IV therapy is essential to prevent this contamination. Although any of the aforementioned antiseptics may be used to cleanse the skin prior to the insertion of a catheter, cannula, or needle, chlorhexidine gluconate is usually preferred. The skin must be gently and thoroughly scrubbed or cleansed with the selected antiseptic solution and then allowed

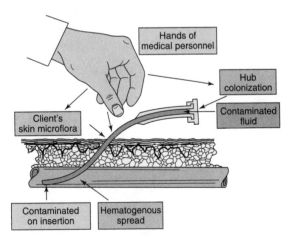

Figure 3-1   Potential sites for contamintion of intravacular device. (From Potter PA, Perry AG: *Fundamentals of Nursing,* ed 6, St Louis, 2005, Mosby.)

to air dry for a minimum of 2 minutes. Once the insertion is completed a sterile dressing is applied to the site. Refer to Chapter 8 for additional information on dressings.

CHAIN OF INFECTION

A factor in the prevention of infection is an understanding of the chain of infection and those factors that encourage the growth of microorganisms (Figure 3–2). For pathogens to be transmitted from one host to another, the following six elements of the chain of infection must be included:

- Causative microorganism
- Reservoir host (source)
- Means of exit from the host (portal of exit from the host)
- Means or method of transmission from the first host to the next host (mode of transmission)
- Means of entrance into the next host (portal of entry into the susceptible host)
- Susceptible host

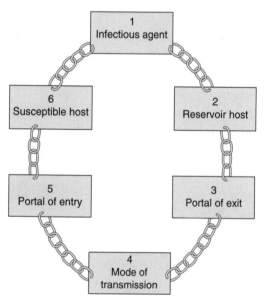

Figure 3-2 Chain of infection. (From Young AP, Kennedy DB: *Kinn's The Medical Assistant: an applied learning approach,* ed 9, St Louis 2003, Saunders.)

Breaking the infection cycle at any point can prevent the transmission of microorganisms that may become pathogens. Frequent hand washing/hand hygiene using proper medical asepsis is essential in health care settings and particularly in initiating IV infusions and caring for existing IV therapy sites. Therefore, continual utilization of medical asepsis in all aspects of care is essential.

Ways to break the chain of infection include the following:

1. For infection to occur, a microorganism with the ability to become a pathogen must be present. Because this pathogen is necessary, breaking the chain of infection before transmission is the best manner to prevent cross-contamination between patients. The growth, reproduction, and survival of causative microorganisms can be halted or impaired by sanitization, sterilization, antiseptics, anti-infectives, or disinfection. The infective agents can be held at bay by depriving them of needed nutrients, thus impairing their potential for growth, reproduction, and survival. Another step in preventing the causative microorganism from surviving and being transmitted to others is to provide appropriate isolation for patients with communicable diseases.

2. The progress of transmission of the microbe from the source host may be blocked, the causative microorganism may be destroyed or reproduction may be prevented, or exposure to the microorganism may be limited. Additionally, it is imperative that health care providers who are ill stay at home rather than appear in the workplace to expose others. Adherence to good hand hygiene and strict sanitization, as well as use of standard precautions and proper disposal of all sharps also is imperative in prevention of the release of the microorganism from the host source. Adhering to the principles of medical and **surgical asepsis** is an essential method of reducing the incidence of transfer of microorganisms from the source host.

3. In the chain of infection, the causative microorganism requires portal of exit from the

reservoir host. Once again, strict adherence to the principles of Standard Precautions, good hand hygiene, use of personal protective equipment (PPE), and proper handling of specimens along with disposal of contaminated articles is helpful in preventing the probability of release of the microorganisms from the reservoir host. Avoiding coughing; sneezing; or talking into another's face, eyes, open wounds, or lesion reduces the risk of spreading the microorganisms.

4. Another means of breaking the chain of infection is to interfere with the method or mode of transmission. Many of the essential guidelines for infection control apply in this aspect of slowing or preventing the transmission of microorganisms. Included is the practice of hand hygiene, strict sanitization, proper sterilization or disposal of used equipment and supplies, good or proper hygienic practices, and avoidance of direct contact with contaminated articles. Other techniques include not allowing items to touch the floor and not shaking linens. Spills should be cleaned and disinfected promptly. When the microbes have no means of traveling to the susceptible host, the chain of infection is interrupted.

5. A portal of entry into the susceptible host is necessary for the chain of infection to continue. Immunizations of healthy potential hosts and isolation of immunocompromised individuals help to protect from the invasion of potential pathogens. Intact skin and mucous membranes are important in the prevention of entry of pathogens. Once again, hand hygiene, proper handling of specimens, proper sharps disposal, and proper disposal of contaminated articles are important steps in reducing the prevention of pathogens entering the host. Additionally, wounds should be covered and any open possible entry sites should be covered or protected. Taking these precautions is necessary to break the transmission of pathogens.

6. A susceptible host, including the very young, the aging population, and those who may be immunocompromised at higher risk, is

necessary for the transmission of the possible pathogen. To interrupt the chain of transmission, these groups of individuals may require extra precaution. Some of the extra precautions include proper nutrition, protective isolation, visitor limitation, and reduction of stress. Proper and frequent hand hygiene, as always, is an excellent tool in preventing the susceptible host from being exposed. Finally, judicious use of antibiotics throughout the years helps to prevent the mutation of antibiotic-resistant pathogens, providing a means of fighting infections that do occur.

Over a period of several years, antibiotics have been prescribed and administered for many minor infections. The individual was not given an opportunity to fight off the invader in a natural way using the person's immunological system. After many **exposures** to antibiotics, disease-causing microorganisms became resistant to antibiotic therapy, developing into "superbugs." Remember, the microorganisms become resistant to the antibiotic, allowing the pathogen to have a greater possibility to be infective. Physicians are now hesitant to prescribe antibiotics for minor infections and encourage the individual's own natural defense system to be allowed the opportunity to fight off the infection. When this is not possible, stronger (or higher generation) antibiotics are used and the potential for new and more resistant microorganisms develop.

MEDICAL ASEPSIS

Medical asepsis, also referred to as clean technique, is maintaining a clean environment and preventing the transmission of disease by reducing the number of pathogens. As previously mentioned, the most important factor and procedure in the maintenance of medical asepsis is proper hand washing technique or good hand hygiene. Additionally, practicing environmental control, following Standard Precautions, using gloves and other PPE, ensuring proper handling of specimens, and disposing of contaminated materials help to halt the exit of the pathogen from its source. Proper disposal of biological waste materials following OSHA's Bloodborne Pathogen Standards helps to ensure medical asepsis.

Cleansing equipment and disinfecting the equipment and surfaces that may have contact with the patient or any instrument or supplies that may come in contact with the patient are means of achieving medical asepsis. To prevent the spread of infection or disease, measures should be taken to destroy any pathogens as they leave the reservoir host. When items are to be used externally on body surfaces, they should be aseptically clean. This is also true of items that may have contact with the surfaces of body cavities that are considered contaminated. An example is the oral cavity or the outer ear. Equipment used on body surfaces should be disinfected after each patient. Stethoscopes should be disinfected after each patient, examination tables should have paper changed and be disinfected after each patient, and any multiuse object or equipment that comes in contact with the patient should be disinfected after each patient. Telephone receivers, mouth pieces, and door handles should be disinfected on a routine basis. The goal is to remove the source of infection from any potential pathogen that has taken up residence in the medical environment. Once again, remember that the first essential step in maintaining medical asepsis is good and frequent hand hygiene.

SURGICAL ASEPSIS

Surgical asepsis, the process that removes all microorganisms, including spores, and is used to maintain sterility of all objects or specific areas, eliminates risks of infection control because the patient is not in contact with pathogens. Sterile technique, also called aseptic technique or surgical asepsis, is required when performing all-invasive procedures, especially when skin integrity may be compromised. Sterilized objects will remain sterile under optimum conditions if not contaminated by breach of sterile procedure during patient care or the supplies are used before the

expiration dates. Sterile procedure is broken when a contaminated or dirty object comes in contact with or crosses a sterile field. The concluding analysis of the comparisons is that the process of medical asepsis reduces or controls the numbers of microorganisms present, whereas surgical asepsis or sterile technique involves the removal of all microorganisms present.

To provide an enhanced understanding of the differences of medical and surgical asepsis a comparison follows:

Medical Asepsis	Surgical Asepsis
1. Kills microorganisms on leaving the body	1. Kills microorganisms before entering body cavities
2. Clean technique with clean equipment and supplies	2. Sterile technique with sterile equipment and supplies
3. Used to prevent the transmission of microorganisms from person to another person	3. Used to maintain sterility when necessary to enter a sterile area of the body
4. Used during noninvasive procedures	4. Used for invasive procedures
5. Hands washed or clean gloves on hands prior to handling any equipment or supplies	5. Hands washed with surgical scrub, sterile gloves worn to handle any equipment or supplies
6. Equipment and supplies are positioned on clean field	6. Equipment and supplies are positioned on a sterile field
7. Protects both the health care professional and the patient	7. Protects the patient undergoing invasive procedures

NECESSITY OF STERILE TECHNIQUE WITH IV FLUIDS

Surgical asepsis or sterile technique is essential in the administration of IV fluids. The process of IV therapy is an invasive procedure in which microbes can enter the bloodstream and the body with ease during any part of the procedure.

Improper cleansing of the skin in the area where the invasive procedure originates can introduce pathogens into an otherwise pathogen-free tissue. A health care provider's improper use of medical or surgical asepsis is another potential source for pathogens to obtain entry into the body.

Allowing the IV tubing to become contaminated creates another source of access for microbes into the body. The infusion site must be kept clean and covered with a secure dressing to prevent entry of microbes. Any time an injection of medication is made into the IV tubing port, sterile technique must be used.

All IV therapy equipment and fluid containers must be inspected for any breach of integrity in packaging. Care must be taken when opening any packaging so that the contents do not become contaminated.

The outer covering or packaging of the IV fluid bag is clean but not sterile. The inner sealed fluid bag is sterile. Once the outer covering is removed, the IV fluid bag will no longer be sterile on the outside unless the clinician who is handling it uses sterile technique. The fluid in the bag remains sterile as long as the integrity of the bag is intact. The same is true of the tubing; it remains sterile on the inside lumen as long as nothing touches either end of the tubing, thus contaminating the inner tubing. The importance in IV therapy is to maintain sterility of the fluids and the tubing throughout the procedure.

USING MEDICAL ASEPSIS TO PREPARE FOR IV THERAPY

In medical aseptic practice, the clinician sanitizes her or his hands with a good aseptic scrub. The IV solution outer wrap is removed and placed on a clean surface and readied for the tubing insertion. The tubing with the protective devices on each end is removed from its packaging and placed alongside the IV fluid container. The catheter or needle is collected and the container is opened, taking care to keep the protective covering in place, leaving the cannula or needle in the package until all supplies are ready.

The tubing is then inserted into the bag port, the bag is hung on a pole or hook, and the tubing is flushed according to guidelines discussed later in the text (see Chapter 8). The selected site should be properly cleansed, and the clinician then dons gloves. After the tourniquet is applied, the needle or cannula is removed from the packaging and insertion into a vein is completed. Once access to the vein is accomplished, the clinician will remove the protective covering and attach the tubing to the needle or cannula hub and secure the infusion and site with appropriate dressing. This process uses medical asepsis. If the process needs to be completed using surgical asepsis, all items handled will be from a sterile field and the clinician will wear sterile gloves.

UNIVERSAL PRECAUTIONS

The Center for Disease Control and Prevention (CDC) established Universal Precautions in 1985 that require all health professionals to follow universal blood and body fluid precautions as a means of reducing the risk of acquiring hepatitis and acquired immunodeficiency syndrome (AIDS) and other bloodborne or body fluid–transmitted diseases (Box 3–1). Universal Precautions classifies all blood, blood products, human tissue, and body fluids as potentially infectious materials. In addition to blood and blood products, semen, and vaginal secretions, body fluids include cerebrospinal fluid, amniotic fluid, joint and other body cavity fluids, and nasal and oral secretions, including saliva.

An additional factor in Universal Precautions is that all health care providers must consider every patient as a potential source of any bloodborne pathogen.

Other guidelines recommended by the CDC for the health care worker include the following:

1. Ensure proper disposal of sources of infectious materials (microbiological waste, pathologic waste, body tissues and fluids).
2. Wash hands before and after gloves are used.
3. Change gloves after each patient contact.

| **Box 3-1** | CDC Guidelines to Decrease Intravascular Infection Related to IV Therapy |

- Palpate catheter insertion site for tenderness daily through the intact dressing.
- Visually inspect a catheter site if client develops tenderness at site, fever without obvious source, or symptoms of local or bloodstream infection.
- Perform hand hygiene before and after palpating, inserting, replacing, or dressing any intravascular device.
- Cleanse skin site before venipuncture with an appropriate antiseptic.
- Do not palpate insertion site after skin has been cleansed with antiseptic.
- Use transparent or sterile gauze dressing to cover a catheter site.
- Replace IV tubing, including piggyback tubing and stopcocks, no more frequently than at 72-hour intervals unless clinically indicated.
- Replace tubing used to administer blood, blood products, or lipid emulsions within 24 hours of initiating infusion.
- There are no recommendations for the hang time of IV fluids.
- Replace dressing over peripheral venous catheters when catheter is replaced or when dressing becomes damp, loosened, or soiled.
- Clean injection ports with antiseptic agent before accessing system.
- Do not use in-line filters routinely for infection control.
- Replace short, peripheral venous catheters and rotate sites every 72 to 96 hours or immediately when complications appear.
- Do not routinely apply topical antimicrobial ointment to the insertion site of peripheral venous catheters or central venous catheter insertion sites.
- There is no recommendation for the frequency of replacement of peripherally inserted central catheter (PICC).

Modified from Centers for Disease Control and Prevention: Guidelines for the prevention of catheter-related infections, MMWR 51(No. RR-10):1-26, 2002.

4. Select and wear personal protective barriers according to anticipated exposure to blood and body fluids. Examples of personal protective equipment or barriers include gloves, face or eye shields, gowns, and masks.
5. Immediately remove protective barriers and thoroughly wash your hands after exposure to blood or other body fluids.
6. Use proper technique when handling, cleaning, and disposing of sharps equipment or supplies.
7. If open or weeping skin lesions are present on provider's skin, patient care should not be provided.
8. Immediately cleanse any blood or body fluid contamination on hard surfaces with 10% sodium hypochlorite solution. Fresh solution should be made daily and not stored because it may deteriorate and lose its effectiveness.
9. Report all sharps injuries immediately. For other CDC guidelines for decreasing intravascular infection related to IV therapy, see Box 3–1. Both the health care provider and the patient may be put at unnecessary risk and may become part of the means of transmission of disease when Universal Precautions are not followed. Strict adherence to Universal Precautions protects the health of medical professionals and patients because some highly pathogenic microorganisms may cause a fatal infection.

Use of personal protective equipment (PPE) is essential when there is a possibility of exposure to **bloodborne pathogens**. Gloves are required and must be properly disposed when removed. Sterile gloves may be required for some procedures but are usually not needed for the routine initiation of an IV infusion. It is prudent to use eye protection or face shields to protect from splashes, spray, or spatters that may occur, especially when starting or discontinuing an IV. Protection for clothing in the form of gowns, aprons, or laboratory coats is suggested.

After initiating IV therapy, disposal of contaminated supplies and equipment must be done according to Occupational Safety and Health Administration (OSHA) guidelines when handling regulated medical waste. Regulated medical waste is any liquid or semiliquid blood, contaminated items that may release blood when compressed, items caked with dried blood, contaminated sharps, and pathological or biological wastes that contain blood. An example is a dressing or surgical sponge that is saturated with blood. This must be disposed in a biohazard bag.

Regulated medical waste must be separated from regular waste items at point of origin. Biohazard containers should be leak-proof and closable. Biohazard bags are to be closed and tied and then double bagged in a second biohazard bag. Biohazard containers must be stored in a secured area that limits personnel with access. Final disposal is regulated by states and usually is contracted with an agency responsible for proper disposal (Figure 3-3).

Sharps include hypodermic syringes and needles; venipuncture needles; lancets; razor and scalpel blades; suture needles; and glassware including blood tubes, capillary pipets, microscopic slides, slip covers, and any broken glassware. Sharps containers must be leakproof, have rigid sides, and be closable. They must be labeled with the biohazard labels (Figure 3-3).

Health care providers initiating or maintaining IV therapy must always use precautions, such as protective gloves, as necessary. Additionally, they should use safety needles when using a syringe and needle. IV needles and cannulas are not safety needles.

OSHA BLOODBORNE PATHOGENS STANDARDS

OSHA, an agency of the federal government, was established in 1970 to guarantee safe working environments for all employees and lower the incidence of occupational hazards. This agency assists employers in providing a safe and healthy work environment for employees. Occupational hazards include possible contact of mucous membrane, skin, or eye or parenteral contact with bloodborne pathogens or other potentially infectious materials.

The OSHA Occupational Exposure to Bloodborne Pathogens Standards were published in 1991. This comprehensive list of regulations, designed to reduce the risk of exposure of employees to infectious diseases, went into effect in 1992.

The Needlestick Safety and Prevention Act was passed by Congress in 2000 to introduce new and safer measures to reduce the number of needlestick and sharps injuries occurring in the health care arena. Safer medical devices were made available, and disposal of all sharps and needles in a safe manner was instituted.

The OSHA Bloodborne Pathogens Standards address the following:
- Exposure control plans
- Labeling requirements
- Safer medical devices
- Record keeping
- Communication of hazards to employees

Medical health care facilities must develop a written exposure control plan that is designed to

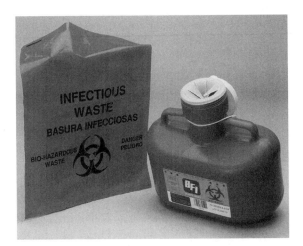

Figure 3-3 Biohazard bag and biohazard sharps container. (From Young AP, Kennedy DB: *Kinn's The medical assistant: an applied learning approach*, ed 10, St Louis 2007, Saunders.)

eliminate or minimize employee exposure to bloodborne pathogens, an obvious danger with IV therapy. The exposure control plan includes the following:

- Exposure determination
- Method of compliance
- Hazards communications
- Infection control practices
- Engineering and work practice controls
- Documentation of training and record keeping
- Postexposure evaluations and follow-up procedures
- Hepatitis B vaccinations.

Finally, training should be supplied to all employees with potential for exposure. They should be provided with a copy of OSHA's Standard for Occupational Exposure to Bloodborne Pathogens. Gloves and other protective equipment are to be readily available, and employees should be instructed on and required to use the PPEs. Training should also include instruction in identification marking and disposal of sharps and blood-soaked material. Management of blood spills is included in training.

Exposure determination identifies employees who must receive training, protective equipment, hepatitis vaccination, and other required protections. All job classifications in which possible exposure might occur are listed, as is the list of job classifications of those who might be accidentally exposed.

Employees also have responsibilities that are also outlined in this act. Any employee with risk of **occupational exposure** to pathogens is mandated to follow these regulations. Those employees must be immunized for hepatitis B, or have the right to refuse immunization and may request the immunization to be administered at a later date without charge. Those declining are required to sign a declination statement (waiver). Employers also must provide training for employees with reference to the control and post-exposure plan. Any clinician initiating or caring for an IV line is at risk for exposure to bloodborne pathogens. It is prudent for these individuals to be vaccinated against hepatitis B.

Those employees at high risk include health care providers such as physicians, physician assistants, nurses, dentists, medical assistants, dental hygienists, surgical technicians, medical laboratory personnel including technicians and phlebotomists, and emergency response personnel.

Needlestick Safety and Prevention Act

Needlestick or sharps injuries must be documented, including a description of the incident (including date, time, and place) and, if possible, identification of the individual whose body substance may have been on the needle or sharp. The clinician should first implement the cleansing and first aid procedure and then report the incident to a supervisor. The employer has the responsibility to obtain consent to test the source's blood as soon as possible for hepatitis B and C viruses and HIV (human immunodeficiency virus). (Some guidelines apply as to source blood; refer to the OSHA guidelines published by the U.S. Department of Labor.) When test results are complete, the injured individual should be notified of the results within legal guidelines. The injured employee should also sign consent allowing for testing of his or her blood as a baseline test. Follow-up testing should be performed within 90 days. If medically indicated, postexposure prophylaxis should be provided to the employee at the expense of the employer.

OSHA and Safety of Patients

Patient safety has been affected by the implementation of OSHA Standards. The risk of pathogen transmission from health care worker to patient has been greatly reduced. Any health care provider who is a known disease carrier and who performs high-risk procedures should be aware of her or his hepatitis B and HIV status. Any health care provider with draining lesions should advise the supervisor; it is recommended that patient contact be restricted.

SUMMARY OF THE NEED FOR ASEPSIS

Sterile technique is an important factor in preventing infections related to intravenous therapy. Medical asepsis is necessary in preventing the chance of infection with the initiation of IV therapy, changing fluids during intravenous therapy, caring for the infusion site, and discontinuing the infusion. The professional has an obligation to be aware of the times for the use of both techniques and must use sterile technique in preparation of the fluids and excellent medical asepsis with the starting of the infusions. For personal and patient safety, Universal Precautions and OSHA Standards should be followed.

Clinicians responsible for initiating, maintaining, and discontinuing IV therapy have a responsibility to the patient and to themselves to practice good hand hygiene and quality infection control. They must follow guidelines for both medical and surgical asepsis. They need to be cognizant of OSHA guidelines and Universal Precautions, and they should practice these concepts and guidelines in patient care. The chain of infection can be broken at any link and infection can be prevented if the clinician uses good aseptic technique. Quality and safe care for the patient is included in the goal of IV therapy.

REVIEW QUESTIONS

1. Compare asepsis and contamination.
2. What is the most important aspect of maintaining medical asepsis?
3. Explain the difference between disinfectants and antiseptics.
4. List three disinfectants commonly used in health care settings.
5. List three antiseptics commonly used in health care settings.
6. List the six elements in the chain of infection.
7. Compare medical asepsis and surgical asepsis.
8. List potential sources of infection as classified by OSHA.
9. Explain the procedure to follow when an accidental needlestick occurs.
10. Why were OSHA's Standard for Occupational Exposure to Bloodborne Pathogens enacted?

Basic Equipment and Supplies for Intravenous Therapy

Chapter Outline

Introduction to Basic IV Equipment

Types of Containers

Types of IV Administration Sets

Types of Needles

Basic Types of IV Solutions

Devices for Regulation of IV Administration

Devices for Holding Infusion Fluids

Supplies for Applying Local Anesthesia before Venipuncture

Supplies for Protection of Infusion Site

Learning Objectives

Upon successful completion of this chapter, the student will be able to:

- Identify and define the equipment needed for initiation of intravenous therapy.
- Identify the types of containers holding intravenous infusion fluids.
- Identify the types of intravenous administration sets and the uses of each type as primary and secondary lines.
- Describe the differences in peripheral or central infusion devices.
- Describe the advantages and disadvantages of needles, over-the-needle catheters, and scalp

- vein or winged needles and the selection for infusion therapy based on patient needs.
- Discuss the basic types of intravenous solutions and the primary uses for each.
- Describe the types of devices used to regulate flow rates of intravenous infusions.
- Decide the adjunct supplies, such as those for dressings, that are needed for safe infusions for patients.
- Describe the safe handling of the equipment and supplies.

Key Terms

back-check valve—device in the primary tubing that prevents the backflow of secondary infusates into the primary line.

bolus—amount of medication given rapidly intravenously that is used to provide a rapid response to the medication or to give a dose to raise the level of the drug in blood.

cannula—sheath used to infuse fluids into the vein.

catheter—hollow flexible tube that is inserted into a vessel or cavity to instill fluids.

collodial—suspension in which small particles are dispersed through the liquid.

crystalloid—solution in which the substances are dissolved in the fluid; a fluid that has the ability to diffuse through a semipermeable membrane.

drip chamber—elongated, enlarged rigid section located at the top of the tubing; holds fluids for administration between the supply container and the tubing.

drop factor—number of drops needed to deliver 1 mL of fluid.

drop orifice—opening in the top of the drip chamber that determines the size and shape of the drop.

flow rate—speed at which IV fluids are regulated for administration.

hypertonic solution—solution that causes a flow of water out of the cell across its semipermeable membrane into the vascular system.

hypotonic solution—solution that causes the flow of water into the cell across its semipermeable membrane from the vascular system.

infusate—parenteral fluid that is slowly introduced intravenously over a specific period.

infusion pump—apparatus designed to deliver a predetermined amount of IV solution or drug through an IV injection over a certain period of time.

injection port—accesses located along primary administration tubing that are used for the administration of secondary infusates.

isotonic solution—solution in which the body tissues can be bathed without the transfer of fluids across the semipermeable membrane of a cell; IV solution with the same tonicity of body fluids.

IV piggyback (IVPB)—set of short tubing that has a standard drop factor of 10 to 20 drops/mL that is added to the injection port of the primary administration set; secondary line for administering infusates over a short time.

macrodrip—tubing that supplies large drops of fluids, such as 8 to 20 drops/mL.

microdrip—tubing that supplies small drops of fluids, such as 50–60 drops/mL.

needleless systems—blunt-tipped plastic insertion device that is inserted into an injection port for the secondary administration of infusates without the use of a needle; the system opens the port and reseals the port on removal.

over-the-needle catheter—infusion set that uses a needle as a stylet and leaves the catheter found over the needle in place for the infusion.

peripherally inserted central catheter (PICC)—long IV access device made of a soft, flexible material that is inserted peripherally and threaded into the superior vena cava.

scalp vein or butterfly needle—infusion needle that has plastic holders on each side of the needle hub to help hold the needle in place during infusion.

spike—sharply tipped plastic end of the drip chamber that is inserted into the infusate container to allow the flow of the infusate from the storage container into the tubing.

stylet—needle or guide that is found within a catheter to allow penetration of the vein and is then removed, leaving the catheter in place.

through-the-needle catheter—catheter that is 8 to 36 inches long and lies within a plastic or metal encasement for the insertion into a vein for IV therapy; the encasement is removed after insertion and the catheter is left in place.

INTRODUCTION TO BASIC IV EQUIPMENT

Types of equipment needed for the infusion of solutions and medications intravenously is based on the needs of the patient, and the proper selection of the equipment to meet the physician's order and patient safety is essential. Through the appropriate choice of the equipment and supplies prior to initiation of the infusion, complications are reduced and problems are minimized during the actual intravenous (IV) infusion. The selection is limited to the choice of IV fluids as ordered, and it is also dependent on the correct decision for flow times based on patient conditions. The patient has little to no input into these decisions, although the safety of the patient is paramount in the correct selection. The person performing the infusion must be sure that patient safety is promoted and that the infusion is effectively delivered.

TYPES OF CONTAINERS

Containers for IV infusions are in open systems, in which the air entering the container displaces the fluids for the infusion, or in closed systems, in which atmospheric pressure is the factor for fluid displacement. In either case, the appropriate infusion sets must be used for the containers to function correctly and to minimize the problems that may occur. When the infusion administration equipment does not match the type of fluid container, the infusion will not be as safe and effective and could even be harmful to the patient.

Rigid or Semirigid Open Containers

Open containers are rigid and usually made of glass, but they are seldom used today except when the fluids to be infused are incompatible with the more commonly used plastic bags. Examples of the incompatibilities include nitroglycerin, insulin, and parenteral lipid additives that cling to the plastic bag.

Glass containers are sealed with a thick rubber disk with an area in the disk for perforation using the tubing **spike** found on the administration set. In this system, air is vented through a filter to allow entrance into the rigid container. This allows fluid to flow by the displacement of the fluids by air. The administration sets may use nonvented sets that have a straw within the bottle. This straw runs the length of the bottle, keeping it above the fluid level to allow air to be pulled in as the fluid is infused. The other type of infusion set for the open containers is a vented set that has a vent at the site of the spike, thus preventing the formation of a vacuum that prevents flow of the fluid.

Glass rigid or plastic semirigid containers provide easy visualization of the fluids in the container, thus allowing the person responsible for the fluids to observe for particles of undissolved medications or other materials that might be floating in the **infusate**. The disadvantages include the possibility of glass breakage during storage or transport, fragments of rubber from the spiking of the container being introduced into the fluids, and the possible contamination from the venting of the fluids. The rigid/semirigid containers also require more storage space and more space for disposal than plastic bags or closed containers. Finally, if the fluids have the rubber disk covering the rubber stopper for spiking removed such as for adding mixtures, the fluids must be used immediately or the opening recovered with a sterile cover immediately following the addition to prevent possible contamination of the sterile fluids or fluid bag.

Plastic or Closed Containers

Most IV fluids today are in closed containers made of flexible plastic. Closed containers are those that do not require venting; instead, the fluids are dispensed by atmospheric pressure. With this system, the bag collapses as the fluids infiltrate and the chance of contamination is reduced because no air enters through the closed system. But, the collapse of the bag on infusion makes the determination of the amount of fluid left in the container difficult to evaluate.

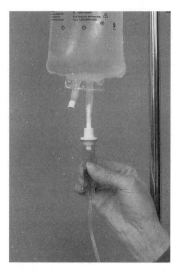

Figure 4-1   Flexible plastic fluid container in closed system. (From Perry AG, Potter PA: *Clinical nursing skills & techniques*, ed 6, St Louis, 2006, Mosby.)

The system is closed to air so the chance of contamination is reduced and the safety for the patient is increased. In these containers, the fluids are easily transported and the chance for breakage is reduced (Figure 4–1). The storage requirements are reduced because the containers are more flexible and weigh less, but the need to inspect the container for possible contamination from tears or leaks is increased. Because of the chance of leaks and puncturing the container, writing directly on the container should not occur.

One of the major disadvantages of the plastic container is the interaction with medications that are added to the fluids. When this interaction with medications has the potential to occur, the use of bags that do not contain DEHP (di-2-ethylhexyl-phthalate, a plasticizer used to make plastic pliable) is indicated. These containers are called semirigid containers—plastic containers that appear to be a bottle. The same needs for venting tubing as found with glass containers are necessary with the plastic semirigid bottles.

With all types of fluid containers, quality control would expect that the person responsible for the infusion should check for clarity of the solution, ensuring that no precipitates are present and that the fluid has not changed color. As with all medications, the expiration date should be checked and any solution out of date should be discarded. If the fluid appears to be contaminated, the container should be so labeled and returned to the proper source.

If the plastic container has been refrigerated, bubbles may be present. In this case, the fluids should be agitated to move the bubbles to the bottom of the bag so these will escape when the bag is spiked and the fluids are primed. Remember that quality control with IV fluids is an important step in patient safety.

TYPES OF IV ADMINISTRATION SETS

Administration sets include the tubing, **drip chamber,** and other accessories to the tubing that are needed to move the fluid from the container to the patient's vein. These sets are supplied in different forms based on the use for the particular patient. The sets vary in the length of the tubing, the size of the drip chamber, and the size of the drops that will be administered per milliliter to the patient. The packaged sets usually contain the **cannula** and needle needed for injection as well as the tubing, whereas other sets allow for the selection of the needle/cannula as separate equipment. In either case, the needle/cannula should be carefully chosen by the responsible person using the needs of the patient, the patient's condition, and the intended use for determining of selection. The infusion sets are labeled individually with the information showing the name; drops per milliliter; the use, such as primary set, secondary set, metered volume set, or other specialty sets; and the gauge/length of the needle/cannula as appropriate. The most frequently used are single line sets that include the primary line and the ability to add secondary lines such as **IV piggyback (IVPB).** In some cases Y-sets are used, as are some specialized sets that will not be included in this basic IV therapy text.

Basic Components Found in Administration Sets

The basic components of administration sets include a spike or piercing pin that is sharply tipped to allow for insertion into the solution container (Figure 4–2). This may be a vented spike as needed for open fluid containers or nonvented sets as needed for closed containers, as described earlier. The spike must remain sterile, so it is manufactured with a removable cover to protect its sterility. The spike has a flange so the fingers do not contaminate the actual spike during the piercing.

The spike is an extension of the **drop orifice** and drip chamber. The drop orifice is found at the top of the drip chamber and determines the size and shape of the drop. These drops are calibrated for the infusion rate in drops per milliliter. This is called the **drop factor** used for calculations of **flow rate**. Primary infusion sets are available in **macrodrip** form, which allows 8 to 20 drops/mL to enter the drip chamber, and microdrip, also called the pediatric chamber, which allows 50 to 60 drops/mL to enter. The **microdrip** or minidrip is used when only small amounts of fluid are to be infused (Figure 4–3).

Tubing connects to the drip chamber and may vary in length depending on whether the set is for primary lines or secondary lines. Primary line tubing ranges from 60 to 110 inches in length, whereas secondary administration sets are between 18 to 70 inches long, with the most frequently used being 30 to 36 inches. The tube varies with flexibility and with internal diameter or lumen. Standard tubing is relatively flexible and is the most frequently used. Macro tubing, used for rapid

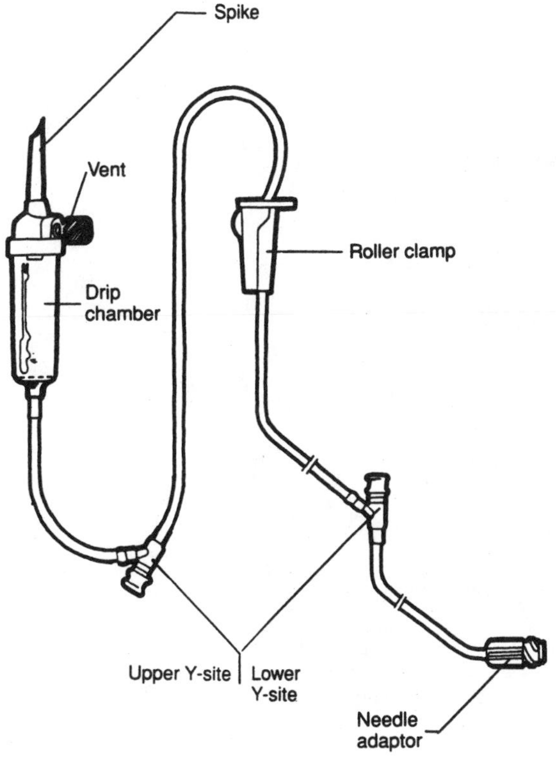

Figure 4-2   Primary administration set. (From Hankins et al: *Infusion therapy in clinical practice*, ed 2, Philadelphia, 2001, Saunders.)

Labels: Spike, Vent, Drip chamber, Roller clamp, Upper Y-site, Lower Y-site, Needle adaptor

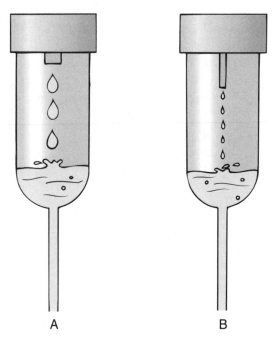

Figure 4-3   A, macrodrip chamber. B, microdrip chamber. (From Clayton BD, Stock YN: *Basic pharmacology for nurses*, ed 13, St Louis, 2004, Mosby.)

flow rates, has a larger lumen and is usually less flexible than standard tubing. Microtubing or microbore tubing is smaller channeled for use with low flow rates, as found with ambulatory infusions of analgesics.

Clamps, injection ports, and **back-check valves** may be found on the tubing, depending on the manufacturer (Figure 4–4). Clamps are used to compress the walls of the tubing to adjust flow rates by changing the size of the lumen of the tubing. The clamp may be on a roller, screw, or slide device, with the slide clamp being the least reliable method of compression. Roller and screw clamps may be adjusted in small increments to regulate the amount of fluid being infused. **Injection ports** are an access into the tubing and are used to add piggyback fluids to the primary set. These ports are usually located along the tubing at various sites, and small-lumened needles or **needleless systems** should be used for the secondary infusion to ensure the port will reseal following the secondary infusion. The backcheck valve is used to allow the primary infusion to continue when the secondary or piggyback

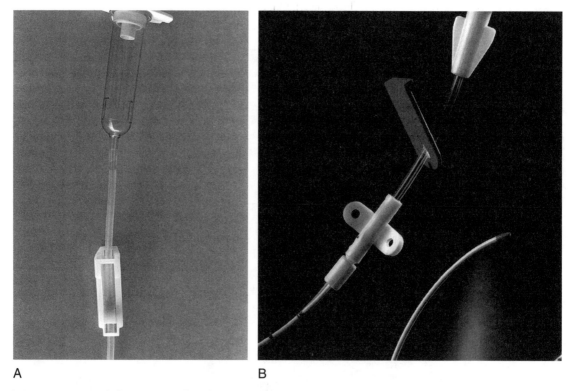

A   B

Figure 4-4   Control clamps. **A,** Roller clamp. **B,** Slide clamp. (**A** from Perry AG, Potter PA: *Clinical nursing skills & techniques,* ed 6, St Louis, 2006, Mosby; **B** from Otto SE: *Pocket guide to infusion therapy,* ed 5, St Louis, 2005, Mosby.)

infusion has completed. It also prevents the secondary infusion from entering the primary solution.

The hub for the needle is the final basic component on the tubing. In most cases, the hub or adapter for the needle will be either a Luer-Lock connector or a slip connection. The slip connection slides onto an IV **catheter** using some force to ensure tightness of the connection and prevent leaks. The Luer-Lock connection requires less force and screws onto the needle or catheter to form a reliable connection against leaks. Luer-Lock connectors are the safest to prevent the accidental disconnection of the needle or catheter from the tubing.

Finally filters may be manufactured in the tubing or may be added to the tubing as needed (Figure 4–5). These filters are used to remove foreign particles such as bacteria, air, particulates, and the like from the infusion prior to the fluid entering the body.

Primary Infusion Sets

Primary infusion sets (Figure 4–2, p. 49) are also referred to as standard sets. These are selected by the correct infusion flow rate and the intended use. The most often used primary infusion set is the nonvented or universal set that is used for plastic bags of fluids. The primary line may also contain

Y-connectors that allow secondary lines to be attached to the primary set. The drop size should be correctly selected for the time of infusion and the condition of the patient. The length of the tubing for the primary set should also be chosen by the size, condition, and ambulatory needs of the patient. The tubing should be long enough to allow the patient some activity while providing for the proper placement and securing of the needed equipment. Therefore, most tubing for primary administration sets is between 60 and 110 inches, usually about 80 inches. Again, remember that the manufacturer's packaging label shows the drop size and the tubing length, and it states whether the tubing is vented and other possible additions to the tubing. In the case where needles or catheters are provided with the tubing, the gauge and length of the needle or catheter will also be shown on the label.

Secondary Administration Sets

The secondary administration set usually has shorter tubing (usually 32 to 42 inches) than the primary set because it is designed to insert into the primary set through the Y-connector or secondary insertion site. A needleless system or a small-gauged needle may be used to insert the secondary lines. When adding secondary sets, the

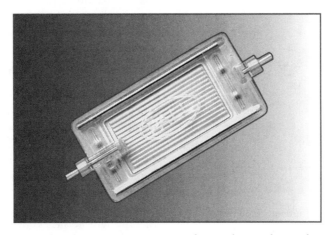

Figure 4-5   Posidyne ELD IV Filter Set. (From Otto SE: *Pocket guide to infusion therapy,* ed 5, St Louis, 2005, Mosby.)

set should either be lower than the container of primary fluids or should have a back-check valve to prevent the back flow of secondary fluids into the primary line (Figure 4–6).

Secondary administration sets are found in two types—piggyback and volume-controlled. The piggyback set has 30- to 36-inch tubing and is used to infuse small amounts of medications. These are used for those patients who are receiving several types of medication therapies simultaneously. The medications, usually in 50- to 100-mL but may be found in 250- to 500-mL, containers, are added to the primary line through a needleless adaptor. When the secondary medication has been delivered, the primary infiltrate resumes infusion. Volume-controlled sets are used when a limited amount of infiltrate is to be administered at a given time. These allow a measured volume of medication to be intermittently administered through a calibrated chamber.

The ports used for secondary administration sets should ideally be punctured using a needleless or needle-protective device to prevent needlestick injuries and to ensure the resealing of the ports

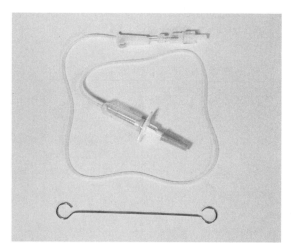

Figure 4-6   Intravenous equipment, including tubing, drip chamber, spike, tubing, flow-control clamp, and Luer-Lock connector. (From Leahy JM, Kizilay PE: *Foundations of nursing practice: a nursing process approach,* Philadelphia, 1998, Saunders.)

following administration of the secondary fluids. Needleless systems consist of a blunt-tipped plastic insertion tool found on the secondary tubing and a port for injection, found on the primary administration set, that opens on activation and immediately reseals when no longer in use (Figure 4–7). The use of this system eliminates the need to use needles and the potential for needlestick injuries, except during the initial insertion of the infusion line.

Adaptors and connectors may be attached to IV administration lines to add more versatility for additions to the lines. These should not be used routinely because each addition to a closed system of infusion has the potential for contamination of the injection port, to the fluids, and thus an increased chance of infection.

Filters may be added to prevent infusion of undissolved solutes, air, or other foreign materials. The filters may be inserted by the manufacturer or may be added through injection ports as appropriate (see Figure 4–5, p. 51).

Stopcocks are used to control the directional flow of the fluids. Available in three- or four-way positions, these are mechanical means of connecting two lines of fluids and provide the ability to administer the desired type of fluid in the desired time. The stopcock will also allow a single type of fluid to be administered at one time or it may allow the combination of the fluids to be infused alternately as needed for a patient's present and ever-changing condition (Figure 4–8).

Central versus Peripheral Infusion Devices

Those persons requiring long-term intravenous therapy may require a venous access line or central venous catheter. There are three types of central venous lines—centrally placed percutaneous catheters, central venous tunneled catheters, and **peripherally inserted central catheters (PICC)** lines that are most often used when intravenous therapy will be necessary for more than a week or will be needed on an intermittent basis over a prolonged period such as with chemotherapy. The catheters are marked with radiographic

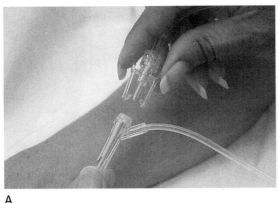
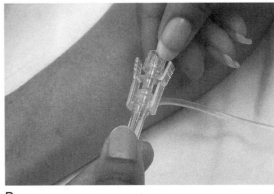

A   B

Figure 4-7   Example of a needleless protective system. (From Perry AG, Potter PA: *Clinical nursing skills & techniques,* ed 6, St Louis, 2006, Mosby.)

materials so the placement can be found using radiography, if necessary. Central infusion devices consist of soft tubing that is more comfortable for the patient and has decreased complications over the long period of time. When long-term venous access, for months up to years, is necessary, these catheters provide patient comfort and decreased complications. Of three general categories of central infusion devices, the physician inserts the centrally placed percutaneous catheters and central venous tunneled catheters, and the PICC may be inserted by other health professionals. These IV access devices are beyond the scope of this text but are mentioned to supply an understanding of IV therapy that is provided over a prolonged period. The routine care of IV lines will be discussed in Chapter 8.

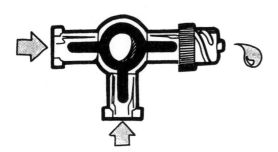

Figure 4-8   Stopcock. (From Hankins et al: *Infusion therapy in clinical practice,* ed 2, Philadelphia, 2001, Saunders.)

TYPES OF NEEDLES

Peripheral infusion insertion devices commonly used for the shorter term therapy include the commonly used **over-the-needle catheters, scalp vein or butterfly needles,** and **through-the-needle catheters.** Through-the-needle catheters are the least commonly used because the needle is used for insertion and then withdrawn and secured outside of the skin. The infusion devices are found in 14 to 25 gauge, with a needle of ½ to 2 inches, and a catheter of 8 to 36 inches in length, if applicable. The catheters are used to deliver viscous fluids and medications. Advantages include less trauma to the veins and greater stability. However, these devices tend to increase the incidence of phlebitis and other infections.

Scalp vein or butterfly needles are frequently used when short-term therapy of less than 24 hours is expected. These devices are excellent for one-time IV medication administration; the needle attaches easily to the tubing (Figure 4–9A, p. 54). The needle size is in odd-number gauges from 17 to 25, with the length varying from 1/2 inch to 1 inch. The plastic wings are attached to the hub and the tubing extends for 3 to 12 inches behind the hub. Because the needles are made of stainless steel and there is the chance of further damage to the veins through accidental puncturing, these devices should only be used for short-term therapy. The use of a needle also increases

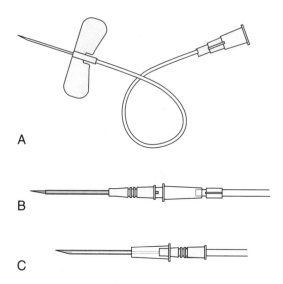

A

B

C

Figure 4-9 Types of needles. **A,** Butterfly. **B,** Over-the-needle. **C,** Through-the-needle catheter (cannula). (From McKenry LM, Salerno E: *Mosby's pharmacology in nursing,* ed 21, St Louis, 2003, Mosby.)

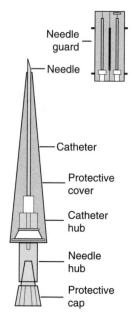

Figure 4-10 Over-the-needle catheter. (From Clayton BD, Stock YN: *Basic pharmacology for nurses,* ed 13, St Louis, 2004, Mosby.)

the risk of infiltration as a result of dislodgement and should not be used where flexion of the extremity might cause dislodgement. Butterfly needles are especially useful with infants, small children, the elderly, and adults with small veins because these cause less trauma to the vein and the blood cells.

Over-the-needle cannulas or catheters consist of a needle with a catheter over the needle. These devices may be found with just the hub or may be found with wings for ease of insertion (Figures 4–9B and 4–10). The needle point, or **stylet,** at the distal tip is used for the insertion of the peripheral device into the vein during the venipuncture. When the blood has flashed back into the hub and the catheter is threaded off the stylet, the stylet is then removed and discarded in a biohazard sharps container. The flexible catheter is left within the vein for the infusion of fluids. The catheter is found in $1/2$ inch to 2 inches in length in gauges of even numbers from 24 gauge to the 14 gauge. Gauges from 14 to 18 are used for major surgery, trauma, or blood administration,

whereas a 20 gauge is most often used with adults. Pediatric patients and adults with small veins would be appropriate for 22-gauge devices. Over-the-needle catheters are easy to insert and stay patent for a longer period of time without the potential of additional trauma to the vein. Infiltration with this device is rare, and the patient has greater mobility because of this stability. The main disadvantage of the over-the-needle catheter is the increased risk for phlebitis.

A through-the-needle catheter is a catheter between 14 and 19 gauge that lies inside the needle and is 1 to 2 inches long (Figure 4–9C). The catheter may be from 8 to 36 inches in length with a steel or plastic encasement that is removed after the catheter has been advanced into the vein. After the catheter is in place, the needle is removed and taped to the outside of the site.

Some catheters are made of thin-walled plastic that allows higher flow rates as a result of the larger lumen. The thin walls also permit the ease of insertion because of the more tapered end at the site of the stylet. The disadvantage is that the catheter has a tendency to lose its shape when it is warmed by body temperature, causing the potential for collapse or kinking of the tubing. Therefore, catheters made of thicker walls have been manufactured. These tend to "pop" on entry into the vein, thus giving the person inserting more confidence of proper insertion. As with other equipment choices, the type of catheter used will depend on what is available and the condition of the patient's veins, as well as the physician's preference.

With any insertion device, the smallest gauge and the shortest length necessary for the delivery of the therapy are the correct choice. Always choose a vein that is large enough for the catheter that can sustain the flow of the IV fluids and blood. Being careful with the choice of veins and size of the catheter will reduce the chance of causing irritation to the vein wall and will decrease the risk of phlebitis.

BASIC TYPES OF IV SOLUTIONS

As previously stated, administration of intravenous therapy falls into three categories—maintenance therapy for meeting the daily needs of fluids; replacement therapy for replacing the losses that have occurred for whatever reason; and restorative therapy for replacing the continued or concurrent losses of body fluids. With these needs for IV therapy in mind, the physician chooses the type of solution that is needed to meet the patient's medical needs. The use of the fluids and the patient's condition will affect the physician's orders and the solutions chosen for infusion.

When the fluids and electrolytes have caused the loss of homeostasis, the most frequent means of replacement is through IV therapy. The physician will evaluate the patient's condition as well as the laboratory tests that indicate the loss of homeostasis. The need for patient safety through the use of the correct type of fluids is of utmost importance. The body will respond to the type of fluid used to provide fluid and electrolyte balance, as discussed in Chapter 2.

Fluids are used to replace vitamins, minerals, and other nutritional supplements when these are added to the basic types of IV solutions. Most fluids administered to the patients on a routine basis are **crystalloid,** meaning that the solutes are mixed and dissolved in the solution so these cannot be distinguished from the actual fluid. These solutes can move through membranes into various body compartments and have the ability to change the character of surrounding tissues. The fluids may be prepared to contain dextrose, sodium chloride, or other electrolytes that have been added by the manufacturer, or the fluids may be specifically prepared for the patient based on the physician's order.

Crystalloid IV solutions are classified as isotonic, hypotonic, or hypertonic. (See Chapter 2 for the effects of tonicity of fluids on body cells and tissues.) For those fluids used to maintain homeostasis see Table 4–1 for the uses and contraindications of each. (For replacement fluids, see Figures 4–11 through 4–17, pp. 57–63.)

Isotonic Solutions

Isotonic solutions are similar to body fluids and are used to expand extracellular fluid space. These fluids do not cause a shift of body fluids in the intracellular, extracellular, and intravascular spaces, but they can be a cause of circulatory overload. Isotonic fluids may also cause a dilution of hemoglobin concentration and may reduce hematocrit levels when given in large quantities.

Simple isotonic IV solutions include sodium chloride 0.9% or normal saline, lactated Ringer's solution, and 5% dextrose in water (Figures 4–11, 4–13, and 4–14, pp. 57–60). These fluids that contain the same amount of electrolytes as found in the body keep the body in a normal steady state and are used to treat patients with fluid loss. Dextrose will prevent the breakdown of chemical compounds in the body, add to the elements for nutritional needs, and provide hydration.

Table 4-1 FLUIDS FOR MAINTAINING HOMEOSTASIS

Common IV fluid	Use	Contraindications
Isotonic saline (0.9%)	Replaces sodium losses in conditions such as gastrointestinal fluid loss and burns	Congestive heart failure, pulmonary edema, renal impairment
Isotonic 5% dextrose in water (D-5-W) Hypotonic 10% dextrose in water (D-10-W)	Maintain fluid intake and provide daily caloric needs, acts as peripheral nutrition, does not replace electrolyte deficiencies	Head injuries, added insulin for persons with diabetes mellitus
Isotonic 5% dextrose in 0.3% NaCl	Supplies calories for nutritional needs	No typical contraindications, added insulin for persons with diabetes mellitus
Hypotonic 5% dextrose in 0.9% NaCl	Maintains fluid intake, is maintenance fluid of choice if no electrolytes are needed	No typical contraindications, added insulin for persons with diabetes mellitus
Isotonic Ringer's solution	Replaces electrolytes in concentrations similar to normal plasma levels, contains no calories	Electrolyte replacement unneeded
Isotonic lactated Ringer's solution	Has similar electrolytes as in plasma, correct metabolic acidosis, replaces fluid losses from conditions such as diarrhea and burns	Congestive heart failure, renal impairment, liver disease, respiratory alkalosis acidosis

From Fulcher EM: *Intravenous therapy: a guide to basic principles*, St Louis, 2006, Saunders.

Hypotonic Solutions

Hypotonic solutions hydrate cells and deplete the amount of fluid in the circulatory system. (See Chapter 2 for the movement of fluids through cell membranes.) With hypotonic therapy, the fluid moves from the vascular system into the intracellular spaces. Less plasma is found in the blood because of the shift of fluids, therefore blood pressure will tend to fall with these fluids. Also, cellular edema will occur if these fluids are not closely monitored.

Hypotonic fluids include 0.45% (Figure 4–15, p. 61) or less of normal saline, dextrose in water of more than 5% concentrations, 5% and greater concentrations of dextrose in normal saline, and 5% dextrose in lactated Ringer's (Figure 4–12, p. 58). Plain sterile water is drastically hypotonic and will not be used for IV infusion except when used as a diluent for medications. Sterile water will affect red blood cells and will lead to lysis of the cells when administered in large quantities.

Hypertonic Solutions

Hypertonic solutions are used to replace electrolytes. Administration shifts extracellular fluids from the interstitial spaces into the plasma for increased blood volume, thus increasing blood pressure. With this shift, severe dehydration may occur, so these fluids should be given slowly and the patient must be closely monitored for circulatory overload. All IV therapy must be watched carefully, but this is most important when hypertonic fluids are being administered. Most hypertonic solutions are for replacement of special fluids and are used for replacement of indicated electrolytes and nutritional elements. These fluids usually have the addition of 5% dextrose (Figure 4–16, p. 62) to raise the hypertonicity of the solution.

Lactated Solutions

Ringer's solutions are isotonic or balanced solutions that are used for rehydration and the replacement of body fluid deficits (Figures 4–15 to 4–17, pp. 61–63). These solutions have electrolyte concentrations similar to extracellular fluids and plasma, so they are effective in the treatment of dehydration from such causes as burns and gastrointestinal symptoms. These fluids do not contain sufficient potassium or calcium for replacement of these losses. Because of the incompatibilities with many medications, the drug should always be checked for safety prior to administration with Ringer's solutions (Tables 4–2 to 4–4, pp. 63–64).

Other Intravenous Fluids

Other specialty intravenous fluids are available for routine maintenance for treatment of such conditions as liver disease, starvation, diabetes, burns, and plasma replacement. These fluids include Plasma-Lyte M, a fluid that has an electrolyte base with the addition of dextrose, to be used for routine maintenance of body homeostasis. Plasma-Lyte R is a replacement solution that provides electrolyte and fluid replacement.

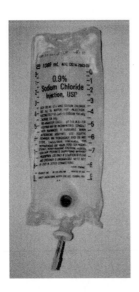

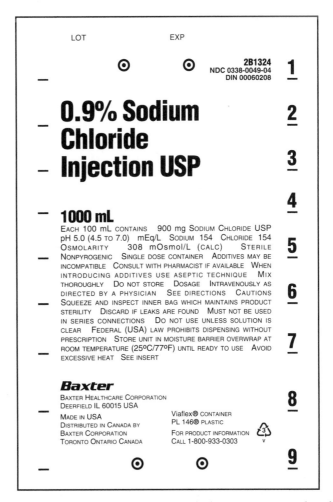

Figure 4-11   Normal saline 0.9%. (From Brown M, Mulholland JM: *Drug calculations: process and problems for clinical practice*, ed 7, St Louis, 2004, Mosby.)

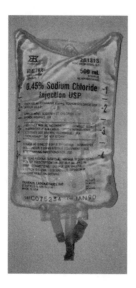

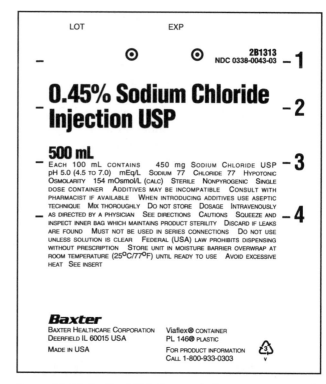

LOT   EXP

—   ⊙   ⊙   NDC 0338-0043-03   **2B1313** — **1**

0.45% Sodium Chloride Injection USP — **2**

500 mL — **3**

EACH 100 mL CONTAINS   450 mg SODIUM CHLORIDE USP pH 5.0 (4.5 TO 7.0) mEq/L SODIUM 77 CHLORIDE 77 HYPOTONIC OSMOLARITY 154 mOsmol/L (CALC) STERILE NONPYROGENIC SINGLE DOSE CONTAINER ADDITIVES MAY BE INCOMPATIBLE CONSULT WITH PHARMACIST IF AVAILABLE WHEN INTRODUCING ADDITIVES USE ASEPTIC TECHNIQUE MIX THOROUGHLY DO NOT STORE DOSAGE INTRAVENOUSLY AS DIRECTED BY A PHYSICIAN SEE DIRECTIONS CAUTIONS SQUEEZE AND — **4** INSPECT INNER BAG WHICH MAINTAINS PRODUCT STERILITY DISCARD IF LEAKS ARE FOUND MUST NOT BE USED IN SERIES CONNECTIONS DO NOT USE UNLESS SOLUTION IS CLEAR FEDERAL (USA) LAW PROHIBITS DISPENSING WITHOUT PRESCRIPTION STORE UNIT IN MOISTURE BARRIER OVERWRAP AT ROOM TEMPERATURE (25°C/77°F) UNTIL READY TO USE AVOID EXCESSIVE HEAT SEE INSERT

Baxter

BAXTER HEALTHCARE CORPORATION   VIAFLEX® CONTAINER
DEERFIELD IL 60015 USA   PL 146® PLASTIC
MADE IN USA   FOR PRODUCT INFORMATION
                        CALL 1-800-933-0303

Figure 4-12 Normal saline 0.45%. (From Brown M, Mulholland JM: *Drug calculations: process and problems for clinical practice,* ed 7, St Louis, 2004, Mosby.)

Dextrose is added to lactated Ringer's to treat burns while replacing electrolyte imbalances.

Other infusions are **collodial** in nature and do not cross membranes because the solutes cannot be dissolved in the solution. Therefore these form a suspension where the molecules are floating for distribution through the liquid. Examples of these specialty solutions are dextran albumin and blood products. Most of these fluids remain in the blood vessels for several days and increase intravascular volume.

DEVICES FOR REGULATION OF IV ADMINISTRATION

IV fluids may be given as an IV push directly into the vein using a syringe at the IV port. This gives a rapid dose of medication, usually timed over 2 to 5 minutes, using a watch to time the medication administration.

When larger doses of medication are needed, this is not a practical means of infusion so the medication may be given by IVPB through intermittent infusions, volumetric chambers, or continuous infusions. With the IVPB, a type of intermittent infusion using a secondary line, the medication is diluted in a small amount of fluids and administered in a drip over a defined period. The timing for administering this infusion must be calculated and the regulation device must be set for the time indicated by the physician's order.

Intermittent infusions are attached directly to an IV lock. This type of infusion also requires the calculation of the flow rate and the proper calibration of the volume control device to ensure

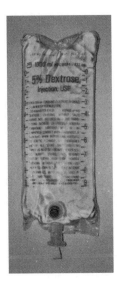

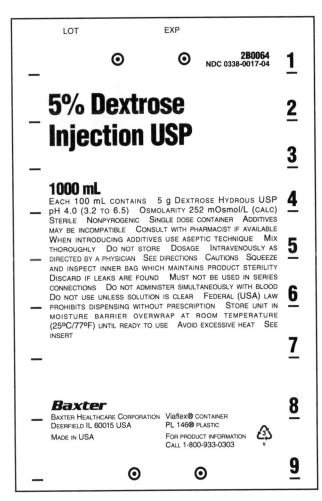

LOT   EXP

2B0064
NDC 0338-0017-04

5% Dextrose Injection USP

1000 mL
EACH 100 mL CONTAINS   5 g DEXTROSE HYDROUS USP
pH 4.0 (3.2 TO 6.5)   OSMOLARITY 252 mOsmol/L (CALC)
STERILE   NONPYROGENIC   SINGLE DOSE CONTAINER   ADDITIVES
MAY BE INCOMPATIBLE   CONSULT WITH PHARMACIST IF AVAILABLE
WHEN INTRODUCING ADDITIVES USE ASEPTIC TECHNIQUE   MIX
THOROUGHLY   DO NOT STORE   DOSAGE   INTRAVENOUSLY AS
DIRECTED BY A PHYSICIAN   SEE DIRECTIONS   CAUTIONS   SQUEEZE
AND INSPECT INNER BAG WHICH MAINTAINS PRODUCT STERILITY
DISCARD IF LEAKS ARE FOUND   MUST NOT BE USED IN SERIES
CONNECTIONS   DO NOT ADMINISTER SIMULTANEOUSLY WITH BLOOD
DO NOT USE UNLESS SOLUTION IS CLEAR   FEDERAL (USA) LAW
PROHIBITS DISPENSING WITHOUT PRESCRIPTION   STORE UNIT IN
MOISTURE BARRIER OVERWRAP AT ROOM TEMPERATURE
(25°C/77°F) UNTIL READY TO USE   AVOID EXCESSIVE HEAT   SEE
INSERT

Baxter
BAXTER HEALTHCARE CORPORATION   Viaflex® CONTAINER
DEERFIELD IL 60015 USA   PL 146® PLASTIC
MADE IN USA   FOR PRODUCT INFORMATION
                                    CALL 1-800-933-0303

1
2
3
4
5
6
7
8
9

Figure 4-13   5% Dextrose. (From Brown M, Mulholland JM: *Drug calculations: process and problems for clinical practice*, ed 7, St Louis, 2004, Mosby.)

the infusion is being administered as ordered (Figure 4–18, p. 64). (Chapter 5 will explain the calculation of flow rates.)

IV medications are added to the volume control chamber by use of a syringe placed in a port on the drip chamber (Figure 4–19, p. 64). These are diluted with the IV solutions that are currently being administered. The timing of the regulation device is set at the length of time necessary for the physician's order with the medication being administered directly into the primary line.

With continuous IV infusion, large volumes of fluids are administered over extended periods, such as several hours to 24 hours. The fluids and any added medications are administered during the entire infusion, and an IV pump or other control device should be used to ensure the proper flow rate for these infusions. In some cases, a fluid time tape may be added to the bag of fluids to give a visual clue that the fluids are being administered over the correct period of time (Figure 4–20, p. 65).

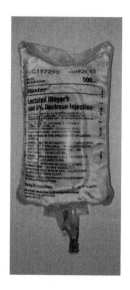 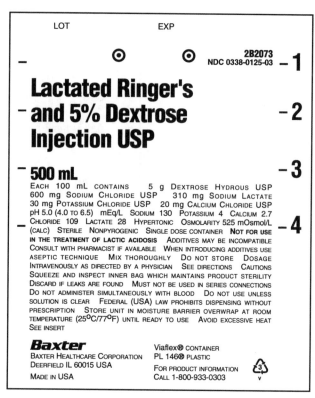

Figure 4-14 Lactated Ringer's and 5% Dextrose. (From Brown M, Mulholland JM: *Drug calculations: process and problems for clinical practice*, ed 7, St Louis, 2004, Mosby.)

Infusion Regulation Devices

With use of IV fluids for patient care increasing and the complexity of drug administration through this route increasing, the use of regulation devices to ensure the correct flow rate for the infusion of fluids has increased dramatically. With the increased need for more control of flow rates, the devices' reliability has increased also. Electronic IV pumps and controllers are designed to precisely measure the flow rate and to regulate the flow at that rate over a period of time. The preselected rate increases patient safety and prevents the accidental changes in flow rates as a result of patient or accidental professional changes. Most pumps will indicate the amount of fluid that has been infused and will automatically prime the tubing prior to the infusion. Some machines today will even indicate where the problems with the infusion have occurred to assist with rapid correction of these problems (Figure 4–21, p. 66). Some devices are much more complicated than others with several channels for simultaneous infusion of different fluids as needed with complex patient care. Others are easily programmed and are even used in the ambulatory care settings (Figure 4–22 A and B, p. 66).

The same rationale for use of regulation devices is found with either the mechanical or electronic devices—to control the rate and to monitor the flow of infusions. Mechanical devices have no power source; rather, they are operated on physical properties such as gravity and the increase or decrease of the flow of the fluids through

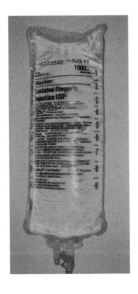

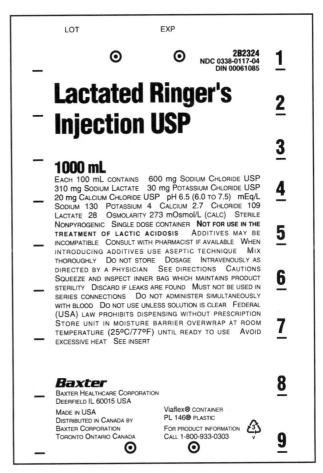

LOT   EXP

2B2324
NDC 0338-0117-04
DIN 00061085

1

Lactated Ringer's Injection USP

2

3

1000 mL

Each 100 mL contains   600 mg Sodium Chloride USP
310 mg Sodium Lactate   30 mg Potassium Chloride USP
20 mg Calcium Chloride USP   pH 6.5 (6.0 to 7.5)   mEq/L
Sodium 130 Potassium 4 Calcium 2.7 Chloride 109
Lactate 28 Osmolarity 273 mOsmol/L (calc) Sterile
Nonpyrogenic Single dose container Not for use in the
treatment of lactic acidosis   Additives may be
incompatible Consult with pharmacist if available When
introducing additives use aseptic technique   Mix
thoroughly Do not store Dosage Intravenously as
directed by a physician See directions Cautions
Squeeze and inspect inner bag which maintains product
sterility Discard if leaks are found Must not be used in
series connections Do not administer simultaneously
with blood Do not use unless solution is clear Federal
(USA) law prohibits dispensing without prescription
Store unit in moisture barrier overwrap at room
temperature (25°C/77°F) until ready to use Avoid
excessive heat See insert

4

5

6

7

Baxter
Baxter Healthcare Corporation
Deerfield IL 60015 USA

8

Made in USA
Distributed in Canada by
Baxter Corporation
Toronto Ontario Canada

Viaflex® container
PL 146® plastic
For product information
Call 1-800-933-0303

9

Figure 4-15   Lactated Ringer's solution. (From Brown M, Mulholland JM: *Drug calculations: process and problems for clinical practice,* ed 7, St Louis, 2004, Mosby.)

the tubing. Electronic devices are powered either by batteries or electrical power to supply the desired flow rate for fluids as ordered.

The most commonly seen mechanical device for regulating the flow rate of fluids is the clamp found on the IV tubing. This method of adjusting the flow rate for infusions is one that has been used for years but is not as accurate as the newer electronic devices. The number of drops per minute must be counted and then calculated to be sure the correct flow rate is being used (Figure 4–23, p. 67). Other mechanical devices include elastomeric balloons made of soft rubberized material that deliver the infusion over a given period. The balloon is inflated to a determined volume of solution so that the medications are delivered at the time predetermined. These may allow delivery over a period of a few hours or may allow delivery over several days. The restriction of the outlet of tubing by the balloon provides safe delivery of the infusion. Spring-coil syringes and containers are other means of mechanical infusion devices (Figure 4–24, p. 68). These types of devices are more often seen in the ambulatory care setting because of the economical factors and the bulkiness of the electronic devices.

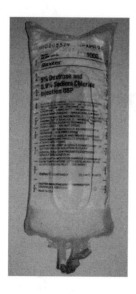

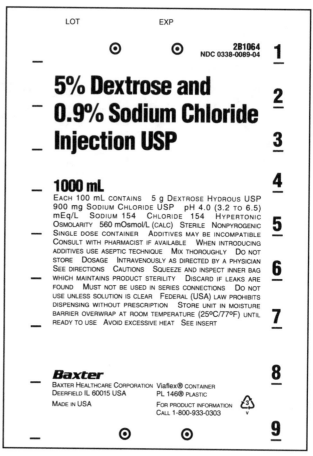

LOT EXP

2B1064
NDC 0338-0089-04

1

5% Dextrose and 0.9% Sodium Chloride Injection USP

2

3

1000 mL

4

EACH 100 mL CONTAINS 5 g DEXTROSE HYDROUS USP 900 mg SODIUM CHLORIDE USP pH 4.0 (3.2 TO 6.5) mEq/L SODIUM 154 CHLORIDE 154 HYPERTONIC OSMOLARITY 560 mOsmol/L (CALC) STERILE NONPYROGENIC SINGLE DOSE CONTAINER ADDITIVES MAY BE INCOMPATIBLE CONSULT WITH PHARMACIST IF AVAILABLE WHEN INTRODUCING ADDITIVES USE ASEPTIC TECHNIQUE MIX THOROUGHLY DO NOT STORE DOSAGE INTRAVENOUSLY AS DIRECTED BY A PHYSICIAN SEE DIRECTIONS CAUTIONS SQUEEZE AND INSPECT INNER BAG WHICH MAINTAINS PRODUCT STERILITY DISCARD IF LEAKS ARE FOUND MUST NOT BE USED IN SERIES CONNECTIONS DO NOT USE UNLESS SOLUTION IS CLEAR FEDERAL (USA) LAW PROHIBITS DISPENSING WITHOUT PRESCRIPTION STORE UNIT IN MOISTURE BARRIER OVERWRAP AT ROOM TEMPERATURE (25°C/77°F) UNTIL READY TO USE AVOID EXCESSIVE HEAT SEE INSERT

5

6

7

Baxter
BAXTER HEALTHCARE CORPORATION Viaflex® CONTAINER
DEERFIELD IL 60015 USA PL 146® PLASTIC
MADE IN USA FOR PRODUCT INFORMATION
CALL 1-800-933-0303

8

9

Figure 4-16 5% Dextrose in normal saline. (From Brown M, Mulholland JM: *Drug calculations: process and problems for clinical practice,* ed 7, St Louis, 2004, Mosby.)

Electronic infusion device controllers allow the fluids to be delivered by gravity, but the photoelectric eye on the tubing monitors the flow rate. The fluid container must be about 36 inches above the IV site for proper flow rates. An alarm sounds when the fluids are not infusing properly. These provide an even, consistent fluid flow so they are safe for use with pediatric or geriatric patients. They are also adequate for use with patients with uncomplicated medical problems.

Infusion pumps use positive pressure to deliver accurate flow rates. The pressure allows the infusion to be accomplished while overcoming resistance caused by excessive tubing length and tape that might be applied too tightly. It is also a means of overcoming resistance caused by viscous fluids, small-gauge catheters or needles, and increased patient activity. The pump has the ability to sense resistance and maintain the IV flow rate by increasing the pressure necessary for fluid delivery. These pumps are especially helpful when positional occlusion by patient movement might occur or when an adjustment in the actual pressure of delivery is desired. Infusion pumps are available for ambulatory use as well as for the inpatient who is essentially on bed rest or is ambulatory for short periods of time. Because of the need to move these devices for patient

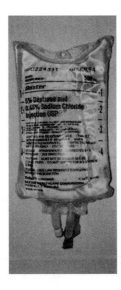

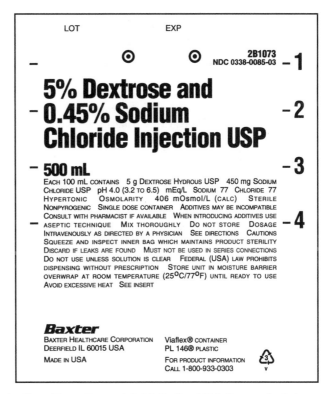

LOT   EXP

NDC 0338-0085-03   2B1073

5% Dextrose and 0.45% Sodium Chloride Injection USP

500 mL

EACH 100 mL CONTAINS   5 g DEXTROSE HYDROUS USP   450 mg SODIUM CHLORIDE USP   pH 4.0 (3.2 TO 6.5)   mEq/L SODIUM 77 CHLORIDE 77 HYPERTONIC   OSMOLARITY   406 mOsmol/L (CALC)   STERILE NONPYROGENIC   SINGLE DOSE CONTAINER   ADDITIVES MAY BE INCOMPATIBLE CONSULT WITH PHARMACIST IF AVAILABLE   WHEN INTRODUCING ADDITIVES USE ASEPTIC TECHNIQUE   MIX THOROUGHLY   DO NOT STORE   DOSAGE INTRAVENOUSLY AS DIRECTED BY A PHYSICIAN   SEE DIRECTIONS   CAUTIONS SQUEEZE AND INSPECT INNER BAG WHICH MAINTAINS PRODUCT STERILITY DISCARD IF LEAKS ARE FOUND   MUST NOT BE USED IN SERIES CONNECTIONS DO NOT USE UNLESS SOLUTION IS CLEAR   FEDERAL (USA) LAW PROHIBITS DISPENSING WITHOUT PRESCRIPTION   STORE UNIT IN MOISTURE BARRIER OVERWRAP AT ROOM TEMPERATURE (25°C/77°F) UNTIL READY TO USE AVOID EXCESSIVE HEAT   SEE INSERT

Baxter
BAXTER HEALTHCARE CORPORATION
DEERFIELD IL 60015 USA
MADE IN USA

Viaflex® CONTAINER
PL 146® PLASTIC
FOR PRODUCT INFORMATION
CALL 1-800-933-0303

Figure 4-17   5% Dextrose in 1/2 normal saline. (From Brown M, Mulholland JM: *Drug calculations: process and problems for clinical practice*, ed 7, St Louis, 2004, Mosby.)

Table 4-2   ADVANTAGES AND DISADVANTAGES OF COMMON FLUIDS

Common Solution	Advantages	Disadvantages
Dextrose in water	Provides carbohydrates, provides nutrition, can be used to treat dehydration	Must be used with care in patients with diabetes
Saline solution	Provides replacement of extracellular fluids, is used to treat patients with sodium depletion	May provide more sodium and potassium than needed, can lead to circulatory overload
Dextrose in normal saline	Can be used to treat circulatory insufficiency, replaces nutrients and electrolytes, is a hydrating solution	May provide more sodium and potassium than needed, can lead to circulatory overload
Ringer's solution	Acts as a fluid and an electrolyte replacement, is a replenisher after dehydration, is similar to normal saline	Can be incompatible with medications, has no calories, causes sodium retention with subsequent congestive heart failure and renal insufficiency
Lactated Ringer's solution	Acts much like extracellular electrolytes	Has no calories, can be incompatible with medications, can increase sodium levels in person with normal sodium levels

From Fulcher EM: *Intravenous therapy: a guide to basic principles*, St Louis, 2006, Saunders.

Table 4-3 AVAILABLE VARIATIONS OF COMMONLY USED FLUIDS

Dextrose in Water	Sodium Chloride	Dextrose in NaCl	Ringer's Solutions
5% Dextrose	0.2% NaCl	5% Dextrose/ 0.2% NaCl	5% Dextrose Ringer's
10% Dextrose	0.45% NaCl (also called $^1/_2$ normal saline)	5% Dextrose/ 0.45% NaCl	5% Dextrose LR (Lactated Ringers)
20% Dextrose	0.9% NaCl (or normal saline)	5% Dextrose/ 0.9% NaCl	
50% Dextrose	3% NaCl		
70% Dextrose	5% NaCl		

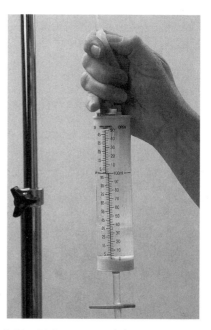

Figure 4-18   Volume control device. (From Perry AG, Potter PA: *Clinical nursing skills & techniques,* ed 6, St Louis, 2006, Mosby.)

Table 4-4 INDICATIONS FOR COMMONLY USED FLUIDS

Solutions	Indications
Dextrose	Maintains homeostasis through sparing the use of body proteins
	Provides basic nutrition of sugars
	Provides calories for energy
	Provides water
	Used as diluent for IV medications
	Treats dehydration
Sodium chloride (saline)	Replaces the loss of sodium and chlorides
	Replaces the lost extracellular fluids
	Used as a diluent for IV medications
	Used to correct water overload of the tissues
	Used to irrigate venous or arterial devices
Dextrose and saline	Hydrates cells
	Promotes diuresis
	Supplies calories
	Used as a plasma extender
	Replaces lost electrolytes and nutrients
Ringer's and Lactated Ringer's	Replaces lost extracellular fluids
	Used to treat burns and dehydration
	Provides electrolytes

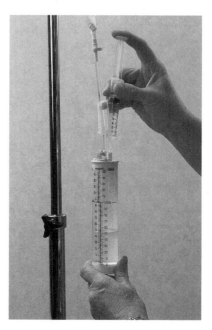

Figure 4-19   Medication injected into volume control chamber. (From Perry AG, Potter PA: *Clinical nursing skills & techniques,* ed 6, St Louis, 2006, Mosby.)

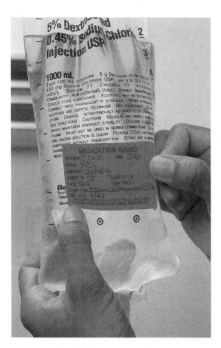

Figure 4-20   Label affixed to IV bag. (From Perry AG, Potter PA: *Clinical nursing skills & techniques,* ed 6, St Louis, 2006, Mosby.)

ambulation, most are found with rollers and have battery power as a means for continuous infusion at the desired flow rate when AC current is not attached.

When using infusion pumps, always follow the directions of the manufacturer because these directions may vary with different pumps, even with the same manufacturer. The drip chamber should be filled to the fill line to allow the sensor to monitor the drip accurately. Alarms indicating malfunction, such as empty infusion fluid containers, air in the line, low battery, and changes in pressure, are available on most pumps used today. The flow rate is adjustable and should be set to the proper calibration and then checked for accurate function at regular intervals during the infusion time. **CAUTION:** Before opening the door on the pump, always clamp the fluids so that the patient does not receive a **bolus** of fluids or medication when the flow rate is not being regulated by the pump.

Remember that pumps vary by manufacturer and style. The person responsible for the infusion should never depend completely on the pump for accuracy of infusion. Rather, the professional should monitor the patient on a regular basis and make the adjustments to the flow rate as indicated to accurately provide the fluids as ordered by the physician. The infusion pump is a device to assist with the proper infusion, but it is not necessarily always accurate. The responsible professional as a routine should check its reliability and monitor the patient for any possible complications. Remember, patient safety is of utmost importance.

DEVICES FOR HOLDING INFUSION FLUIDS

Poles for holding IV fluids are available in various styles including those freestanding on the floor or poles that attach to either the patient bed, chair, or gurney to allow for transportation or ambulation of the patient during infusion therapy. In some settings a device may be attached to the ceiling with hanging loops used to hold the IV fluid container. Loops may also be used to hang fluids at different levels above the patient to allow for different infusion rates of designated fluids (see Figure 4–6).

Some IV poles are designed to be relatively lightweight and portable, whereas others are heavy duty for holding several containers of fluids, monitors, and other needed devices. The needs of the patient and the location of the patient during the infusion determine the type of device needed for holding the IV infusates and the necessary ancillary equipment for patient care.

SUPPLIES FOR APPLYING LOCAL ANESTHESIA BEFORE VENIPUNCTURE

In some instances a local or topical anesthetic is used prior to the insertion of the venipuncture device. If the area to be injected is in a very sensitive area of the body, more advanced

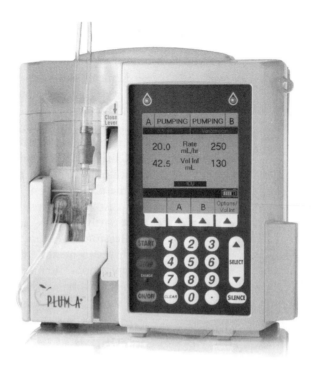

Figure 4-21   Abbott Plum A infusion pump. (Courtesy Abbott Laboratories, Abbott Park, Ill. From Otto SE: *Pocket guide to infusion therapy*, ed 5, St Louis, 2005, Mosby.)

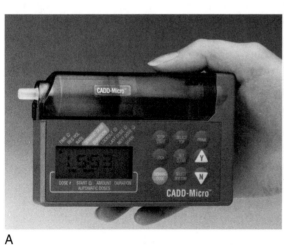

A

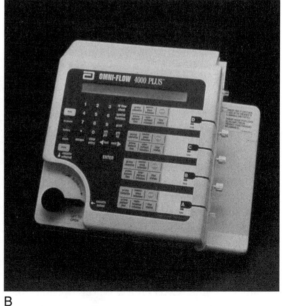

B

Figure 4-22   **A,** CADD-Microambulatory infusion pump, model 5900. **B,** Omni-Flow 4000 Plus infusion pump. (**A** courtesy SIMS Deltec Inc., St Paul, MN; **B** courtesy Abbott Laboratories, Abbott Park, IL. From Otto SE: *Pocket guide to infusion therapy*, ed 5, St Louis, 2005, Mosby.)

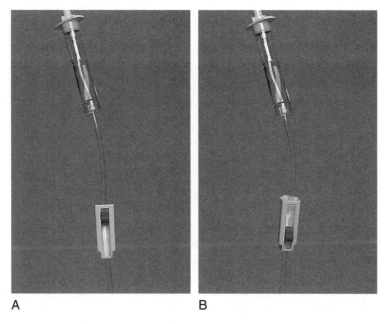

A   B

Figure 4-23   **A,** Roller clamp in open position. **B,** Roller clamp in closed position. (From Perry AG, Potter PA: *Clinical nursing skills & techniques,* ed 6, St Louis, 2006, Mosby.)

level of anesthesia, such as a nerve block, may be used.

Topical anesthesias are used to prevent the pain of the insertion of the venous access device by providing anesthesia directly over the vein site. The two most often used topical local anesthetics are EMLA and ELA-max, which are **eutectic mixtures** of local anesthetics. EMLA is a nonsterile emulsion of 2.5% lidocaine and 2.5% prilocaine that is thickened to the consistency of a cream but becomes oily at room temperature or when applied to the skin. Absorption is more effective on the thin epidermal area rather than on the thicker epidermal sites. The duration of action is approximately 1 hour, and the depth of anesthesia is 5 to 6 mm. ELA-max is essentially the same medication except that it contains 4% lidocaine in a special delivery system that provides greater anesthetizing power to the area. These topical anesthetics should not be applied to open areas of the skin; they should only be applied directly to the proposed area for the infusion. These should be applied at least 5 minutes prior to the venipuncture but are more effective if left in place for longer periods of time prior to insertion of the venipuncture. The skin should not be cleansed with alcohol or other cleansers prior to use because the natural body oils seem to enhance the effectiveness of EMLA and ELA-max. EMLA should have an occlusive dressing applied over the mound of medication to hasten anesthesia; ELA-max does not need the dressing, but a covering may be applied to reduce the oily mess that occurs following application.

Intradermal local anesthesia may also be used in those instances where the time needed for topical anesthetics is not available. The injection or infiltration of the medication, such as lidocaine in various strengths, is accomplished at the site of the IV insertion. This is a safe, effective, and economical means of providing anesthesia, although the discomfort of injection of

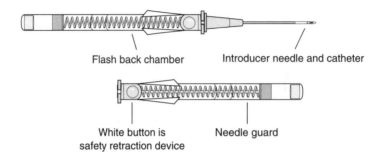

Figure 4-24 Spring-coil syringe. (From Perry AG, Potter PA: *Clinical nursing skills & techniques,* ed 6, St Louis, 2006, Mosby.)

the anesthetic is present. The burning from the local anesthetic may last up to 15 minutes following injection and is one of the major drawbacks to this type of local anesthesia. A small-gauged needle (25 to 29 gauge) is used for the injection of approximately 0.1 to 0.3 mL of anesthetic. As with all intradermal injections, the bevel of the needle will be placed upward, allowing the formation of a wheal. If need be, the wheal may be compressed to allow the diffusion of the anesthetic into the area.

Use of local anesthetics prior to insertion of the IV needle or catheter is a safe and effective way to reduce the pain associated with venipuncture. It can be used with patients with low pain thresholds, in pediatric and geriatric patients, and in circumstances where replacement of the infusion is necessary.

SUPPLIES FOR PROTECTION OF INFUSION SITE

Dressing materials for infusion sites vary with the location of the dressing, the needs of the patient, and the protocol of the location of employment. The Centers for Disease Control and Prevention (CDC) states that all dressings at the infusion site should be sterile. The materials used are found in two categories that range from gauze and tape to specialized semipermeable materials that are occlusive. The timing for

changing dressings is controversial, although most protocol states that all gauze and tape dressings should be changed every 48 hours or before if the integrity of the dressing has been compromised. When these dressings are applied, the tape for securing the dressing should be marked with the date and time of the application and it should be initialed by the person who changed it.

Sterile gauze used for these dressings should be lint-free so it will not adhere to the site. Lint adhering to the site will hinder healing and could be a cause of infection. If the gauze is used for absorption, the cotton material may be the best, but if the gauze is for padding of the site, the material would preferably be a synthetic. The gauze dressing is less expensive but has the disadvantage that the infusion site is not visible for a regular inspection. If the gauze dressing is lifted to inspect the site, new dressing should always be applied.

Semipermeable membrane dressings are transparent and allow for the visualization of the infusion site. These individually packaged sterile dressings are designed to allow the moisture from the skin to be drawn through the dressing to prevent excess moisture on the skin. The rate at which the moisture is released varies by manufacturer and the product, but even the best of these dressings are vulnerable to release from the skin as a result of perspiration and wound drainage. These dressings should not be allowed to remain in place for more than 72 hours, with the length being determined by the protocol of the institution of practice. As with other dressings, these should indicate the date and time changed. In most instances, the dressing and the infusion site should be changed at the same time. The skin should be dry at the time of application, and no ointment or any other greasy substance should be used near the dressing application site. When applying the semipermeable membrane dressing, it should cover the insertion site and then should be pinched around the catheter or needle hub to secure the hub and tubing to the skin. Finally the insertion site should be labeled on a piece of adhesive tape that is not placed directly over the transparent dressing, with the catheter gauge, date and time of insertion catheter, and the initials of the person who performed the venipuncture or dressing change. If only the dressing is changed, a note should be made of the date and time of the original venipuncture If the adhesion of the dressing is impaired prior to the time to change the entire IV infusion site, the sterile dressing should be applied to the cannula hub and wings of the infusion set. The transparency of the dressing allows the constant inspection of the site and the dressing is more comfortable for the patient. Although these are more expensive than gauze and tape, a major advantage of these dressings is that the patient will be able to bathe without saturating the dressing.

Antimicrobial patches are available and may be applied under the dressing or used alone. The patch contains chlorhexidine to reduce bacterial contamination and is smaller than the other dressing materials. Each patch, with a precut slit for the application around the infusion set, is smaller than a regular dressing but is also absorptive, nonirritating, and nontoxic. Use of these patches is particularly indicated with persons with increased susceptibility to infections.

The equipment and supplies for IV therapy must be carefully handled at all times. The equipment and supplies that come in direct contact with the IV infusion site and the fluids administered must be kept sterile at all times. Some supplies must be kept aseptically clean for the protection of the patient against infection. The protocol of the site of employment should always be followed with the professional using the supplies taking great care in ensuring patient safety is of utmost importance.

REVIEW QUESTIONS

1. What are the three types of container in which IV fluids are supplied?
2. What are the advantages of the plastic bag of fluids over glass containers?
3. What are the major disadvantages of plastic bags of fluids over glass containers?
4. What are the three major types of devices used to initiate an IV infusion?
5. Why are catheters or cannulas preferable to needles for IV infusions that will last longer than a few hours?
6. Why are needleless systems the preferable means of adding secondary lines of IV administration to primary lines?
7. What are the four most commonly used types of IV fluids?
8. What are the primary uses of saline solutions?
9. What does dextrose in fluids supply?
10. Why are infusion pumps preferable to the use of clamps on IV lines in regulating flow rates of fluids?

5
Review of Dosage Calculations

Chapter Outline

Calculating Dosage Using the Metric System

Calculating Basic Dosage

Interpreting IV Fluid Labels

Calculating Solute Weights during Infusion

Calculating IV Flow Rates

Calculating IV Infusion Times

Calculating the Amount of a Drug in a Solution

Calculating the Amount of Medication Infused in the Amount of Fluids

Calculating IV Medications in Amounts per Kilogram of Body Weight

Learning Objectives

Upon successful completion of this chapter, the student will be able to:

- Identify the weight and volume measures of the metric system.
- Calculate the basic dosages related to the administration of IV medications, including percentages of solvents in standard IV fluids.
- Interpret the meaning of abbreviated labels for common IV fluids.

- Calculate drip rates of IV fluids.
- Calculate flow rates of IV fluids.
- Calculate infusion times of IV fluids.
- Identify factors that might influence the flow rate of IV fluids.

Key Terms

cubic centimeter (cc)—one centimeter cubed; equivalent of 1 mL.

flow rate (FR)—speed at which IV medications are infused.

gram (g, gm, G, Gm)—basic measure of weight in metric system.

liter (L)—basic fluid measurement in the metric system.

metric system—decimal system of measurement based on liter for fluids, gram for solids, and meter for length.

milligram (mg, mG)—one thousandth of a gram.

milliliter (ml, mL)—one thousandth of a liter.

percentage—parts per hundred.

solute—substance dissolved in a solution or semisolid.

solvent—substance in which a solute is dissolved, either a liquid or semisolid.

volume of medications—fluid amount of a medication.

weight of medications—solid amount of a medication.

As health care professionals the calculation of medications is not a new concept and probably is one that is used daily in your professional life. In this chapter we will review the basic concepts of **weight** and **volume** of the metric system because these are used with intravenous (IV) therapy. The basic calculations using the formula method and ratio/proportion will be included. After the physician has ordered the fluids for the patient, the correct **flow rate (FR)** to be used for administering the fluids during a specific time, such as a minute or hour, must be calculated. This calculation ensures that the order is accurate and that it will be safe for the patient. This chapter is intended to facilitate the calculations that may have been used in times past but have not been recently practiced. The hope is that the review will be a means of recalling knowledge previously gained.

The preparation of the fluids to be administered may be done by the person performing the administration, or these fluids may be prepared in a pharmacy prior to administration. When the pharmacy is involved in preparation, the triangulation between the health professionals—the physician who orders the fluids, the pharmacist who prepares the fluids, and the health professional administering the fluids—provides an added degree of patient safety. Through the entire process the verification of the order and the correct patient as well as the administration using the correct dose, time, rate, and route are necessary prior to administering the fluids.

CALCULATING DOSAGE USING THE METRIC SYSTEM

The **metric system** is the universally used system of measurement and the system most often used in the medical field. Because medications that are administered intravenously are immediately in the bloodstream for absorption, the exact dosage of a medication as ordered by the physician must be calculated and administered. Therefore, most medications are found in metric dosages and

the metric system will be used often when administering any medications, including those given by infusion.

The metric system provides many of the commonly used dosage indications in both weight and volume measurements. The weight measurements in the metric system are determined using the base **gram (g or gm)**. The increments are in magnitudes of 10 from kilograms (kg) being 1000 grams to micrograms (mcg or μg) being 1,000,000th of a gram. The main metric weights used for dosage calculations are gram, **milligram (mg),** microgram, and occasionally kilograms. Volume measurements in the metric system are in increments of 10 with a base of **liter (l or L)**. The most commonly used volume measurements for liquid medications, including IV fluids, are **milliliters (ml or mL)** and liters, with liters containing 1000 mL. Remember that a milliliter may also be called a **cubic centimeter (cc)** because these both occupy the same amount of liquid space. The length measurements of centimeter (cm) or millimeter (mm) are seldom used with calculations for IV fluids.

Because the metric system is based on units of 10, decimals are used to show and calculate fractional amounts of medication. To convert a dosage amount to the next smaller unit, the decimal is moved one place to the right. Conversely, when moving from a smaller unit to the next larger unit of the metric system, the decimal is moved one place to the left. In the medical field, most conversions are made in 1000 units rather than in 10 units, so the decimal will be moved three places in most equations. For example, a gram is larger than a milligram so to change 1 gram to milligrams, the decimal is moved three places to the right and three zeros are added to show that 1 gram equals 1000 milligrams.

1 gram = 1 g or to move to milligrams 1 g = 1000 mg

Likewise, 1 milligram = 1 mg or to move to micrograms, 1 mg = 1000 mcg.

To convert from 1 liter to milliliters, the same movement to the left is necessary or

$$1 \text{ L} = 1000 \text{ mL}$$

However, to move from 1 g to kilograms, the movement is to the left and the decimal is moved behind the kilogram. 1 g = 0.001 kg

The metric system is shown in decimals because it is based on units of 10 (Table 5–1). To prevent medication errors when using the decimal system, always be sure that if a medication dose is a number less than one designation, a "0" should always precede that decimal point to prevent miscalculation of the dose to be given. Never allow a decimal point to be the first unit in a dosage indication (i.e., .025 mg should be shown as 0.025 mg or 25 mcg).

Learning Note

Always remember that the metric system is based on measurements of 10 between each designation. A kilogram to gram is a proportion of 1000 and a gram to a milligram is another 1000 proportion as is milligrams to micrograms. The proportion is the same for milliliter to liter.

CALCULATING BASIC DOSAGE

Determining doses of medications is a basic task for medical professionals. This may be accomplished by using either ratio/proportion (*DA [Dosage Available]: DF [Dosage Form]:: DO [Dose Ordered]: DG [Dose to be Given]* or by using the formula method (*DD [Dose desired]/ DH [Dose on hand] × Qty [Quantity or form] = Dose to be given)*. With the ratio/proportion method, the means (the two numbers next to the equal signs or ::) should be multiplied by each other and the same for the extremes (the two numbers on the outside of the equation). When using ratio/proportion, the calculated answer should always be checked because following calculation the final answer of the multiplication of the means

Table 5-1 METRIC CONVERSION FACTORS

Metric Weight Volume
1 kg = 1000 g
1 g = 1000 mg
1 L = 1000 mL (cc)
1 mg = 1000 mcg
1 mcg = 0.001 mg
1 mg = 0.001 g
1 mL = 0.001 L

should equal the final answer of the multiplication of the extremes. The answer of the calculation will be in the designation of "x." For example, if the equation mg: mL = mg: mL is used and the x is in the placement of the milliliter, the answer will be in milliliters. Always insert the "known" designations in the first ratio, being sure that all designations are within the same measurements systems. Also be sure that the like components in both ratios are in the same weight or liquid measure (i.e., mg in one ratio must be mg in the second ratio, not g or mcg). If the components are not the same, conversions within the system must be made prior to calculating the dosage.

EXAMPLE: A physician orders ampicillin 500 mg q6h to be infused to a patient with acute bronchitis. The medication is available as 1 g/4 mL following reconstitution. What volume of medication should be supplied to the patient every 6 hours?

Before the calculation can be made, the weight of the medication must be in the same metric measurement. One g is equal to 1000 mg. This should be changed to milligrams because this is the weight used in the order.

Ratio/Proportion Method

1000 mg (DA): 4 mL (DF):: 500 mg (DO): x (DG)

$$1000 \text{ mg} \times x = 4 \text{ mL} \times 500 \text{ mg}$$

$$1000 \, x = 2000 \text{ mL}$$

$$x = 2 \text{ mL}$$

Formula Method

$$500\text{mg}/1000 \text{ mg} \times 4 \text{ mL} = \text{Qty}$$

$$\frac{500 \cancel{\text{mg}}}{1000 \cancel{\text{mg}}} \times 4 \text{ mL} = \text{Qty}$$

$$\frac{1}{2} \times 4 \text{ mL} = \text{Qty}$$

$$2 \text{ mL} = \text{Qty}$$

INTERPRETING IV FLUID LABELS

When interpreting the fluids that the patient is to receive, the commonly used infusates are available in **percentage** strengths in specific fluid amount. The first letter indicates the chemical that will be found in the fluid, the second number is the percentage strength of that chemical, and the third designation is the fluid in which the chemical is found. When a label reads 1000 mL NS it indicates that 0.9% sodium chloride (NaCl) or normal saline in 1000 mL containers. This designation actually means the parts per hundred of the **solvent** (NaCl) in the **solute** (water). In this example, the use of percentage states that 0.9 g of NaCl is found in each 100 mL of solute (usually water) or 9 g of NaCl are found in 1000 mL of solute or water. Another example of the use of percentage of solute in solvent is 5% dextrose in $^1/_2$ NS (D-5-1/2 NS). In this case, 50 g of dextrose and 4.5 g of NaCl ($^1/_2$ NS indicates that the NaCl is 0.45% rather than the 0.9% found in NS) would be found in each 1000 mL of water. (Remember, the percentage amount is in 100 mL, NOT 1000 mL, so the percentage amount must be multiplied by the number of milliliters in the container.) Understanding the percentage of solute in a solvent is important for patient safety when administering fluids. When choosing the correct fluids for the patient, be sure that the percentages agree with the physician's order.

Learning Note

1 mL of water used as a solvent weighs the same as 1 g of solute.

This information is just a reminder of the necessary background for administering medications and fluids. In most cases when drugs are added to IV fluids, this is accomplished by a pharmacist so the actual calculation and preparation of the medication dose has already been done. However, the person infusing the medication has the responsibility of being sure that an accurate dosage has been calculated and prepared. Therefore, all fluids administered with medications added should be rechecked for the accuracy of preparation and should be checked to the physician's order prior to hanging the infusate. Again, the triangulation between health professionals provides quality assurance for patient safety.

CALCULATING SOLUTE WEIGHTS DURING INFUSION

The understanding of percentage of solutes in solvents is essential as the patient is monitored during the infusion. The total chemical content of infusates will affect how the patient reacts to the IV fluids, and early intervention of possible adverse reactions may be possible if the percentages of electrolytes and chemicals being used are known. Consider the person with diabetes mellitus who is receiving IV fluids with dextrose. The amount of dextrose will certainly be a factor in the patient's response to the IV therapy. Remember that once IV fluids are injected into the vein, these medications cannot be retrieved, so care for understanding percentages of solutes in solvents is essential.

In some cases, a physician may ask that the amount of solute be calculated when the entire fluid amount is not infused. For example, a patient may have an order for 500 mL D-5-NS (5% dextrose in 0.9% sodium chloride). The fluids infiltrate after the patient has received 300 mL. How many grams of dextrose and how many grams of sodium chloride did the patient receive?

The way to calculate the weight of solutes is by using ratio/proportion:

Known   Unknown

25 g dextrose (5 g/100 mL): 500 mL:: x g: 300 mL

$$500 \, x = 7500 \text{ g}$$

$$x = 15 \text{ g dextrose}$$

Known   Unknown

4.5 g NaCl (0.9 g × 500 mL): 500 mL:: x g: 300 mL

$$500 \, x \text{ g} = 1350$$

$$x = 2.7 \text{ g}$$

So if the patient received 300 mL of D-5-NS, the total amount of dextrose infused is 15 g and the total amount of NaCl is 2.7 g.

CALCULATING IV FLOW RATES

Fluids may be infused without added medications, but in many instances the medication is added for therapeutic reasons. The physician's order for the rate of administration of the fluids will vary depending on the condition of the patient and the medications or fluids that are to be infused. The physician's order may state the number of milliliters per minute the patient should receive, whereas in other cases the physician may designate the time that is needed for the infusion.

The calculation of drops per milliliter is called flow rate, a mathematic problem that is dependent on the equipment that has been chosen for use. Remember from Chapter 4 on equipment that the administration set may be designated as either a macrodrip set that provides the fluids in 10 to 20 drops per milliliter or a microdrip set that provides 50 to 60 drops per milliliter. Remember that the size of the drop is basically determined by the drop size into the drip chamber. The macrodrip is used for adults in most instances, whereas the microdrip sets (sometimes abbreviated as µgtt or called the pediatric chamber) often are used in pediatric patients, or with

persons or medications that require small amounts of medication fluids per time period.

The rate of flow or the infusion rate in drops is also dependent on the amount of pressure on the tubing, whether this is from a clamp device or from an infusion pump. Before any calculations of the flow rate can be performed, the size of the drop from the label of the administration set as provided by the manufacturer must be known. This information is found on the box of the administration set—so the correct administration set must be carefully chosen to meet the physician's order. This drop factor will be used for the infusion flow rate. If there is a doubt after the administration set is in place, the tubing also contains the information concerning the drop factor. Also, remember that the attached tubing is not interchangeable with other drip chambers because the lumen of the tubing has also been considered with the drop factor.

The four factors to be considered with the administration of fluids are as follows:
1. The total amount of fluids to be administered in milliliters
2. The calibration of the administration set in drops/milliliter (gtt/mL)
3. The flow rate of the fluids in drops/minute (gtt/min)
4. The time for the fluids to infuse in minutes (min)

EXAMPLE USING FORMULA METHOD: When the amount of fluid, the calibration of the administration, and the time for fluid infusion are known, the rate of flow or the time for infusion can be calculated using the following formula:

$$\text{Flow rate} = \frac{\text{Amount of fluid} \times \text{Calibration on administration set}}{\text{Time for infusion (minutes)}}$$

OR

$$\text{Flow rate} = \frac{\text{mL ordered} \times \text{gtt/mL (drop factor)}}{\text{min for infusion (Time for infusion)}}$$

EXAMPLE: A physician orders 1.5 L of lactated Ringer's to be infused over 8 hours. The infusion administration set reads 20 gtt/mL

$$\text{Flow rate} = \frac{1500 \text{ mL} \times 20 \text{ gtt/mL}}{8 \text{ hr} \times 60 \text{ min/hr}}$$

(The hours must be changed to minutes because the formula indicates minutes for infusion. Liters must be changed to milliliters to match the administration set that is designated in milliliters.)

$$\left(\text{Dividend is: } \frac{1500 \text{ mL} \times 20 \text{ gtt}}{1 \text{ mL}} \right)$$

$$\left(\text{Divisor is: } \frac{8 \text{ hr} \times 60 \text{ min}}{1 \text{ hr}} \right)$$

$$\text{Flow rate} = \frac{1500 \times 20 \text{ gtt}}{8 \text{ hr} \times 60 \text{ min}} = \frac{3000\emptyset \text{ gtt}}{48\emptyset \text{ min}}$$

$$\text{Flow rate} = \frac{3000\emptyset \text{ gtt}}{48\emptyset \text{ min}}$$

Flow rate = 62.5 gtt/min or 63 gtt/min.

If it is easier for you to complete the infusion rate in two steps, the following two steps may be used:

EXAMPLE: A physician orders 1.5 L of lactated Ringer's to be infused over 8 hours. The infusion administration set reads 20 gtt/mL.

Step One:

$$\text{mL/hr} = \frac{\text{Total volume of fluids(TV)}}{\text{Total time in hours(TTH)}}$$

$$\text{mL/hr} = \frac{1500\text{mL(TV)}}{8\text{hr(TTH)}}$$

mL/hr = 187.5 or 188 mL per hour should be administered

Notice that the problem at this point is milliliters per hour. Now the time should be

converted to minutes because the flow rate will be in drops/minute.

Step Two:

$$\text{gtt/min} = \frac{\text{Drop factor (gtt/mL)}}{\text{Time in min (TM)}} \times \text{Total volume per hour}$$

$$\text{gtt/min} = \frac{20 \text{ gtt/mL}}{60 \text{ min}} \times 188 \text{ mL/hr}$$

$$\text{gtt/min} = \frac{\overset{1}{20} \times 188}{\underset{3}{60}}$$

$$\text{gtt/min} = \frac{188}{3}$$

gtt/min = 62.7 or 63 gtt/min

EXAMPLE USING DIMENSIONAL ANALYSIS: If dimensional analysis is the preferred means of calculating dosage, the following is the manner for calculation.

A physician orders 1.5 L of lactated Ringer's to be infused over 8 hours. The infusion administration set reads 20 gtt/mL.

The formula needed to use dimensional analysis is as follows:

$$\text{DF} \times \text{CFV} \times \text{DV} \times \text{DT} \times \text{CFT} = \text{FR (flow rate in gtt/min)}$$

DF = Drop factor (gtts/mL)
CFV = Conversion factor volume (mL/L)
DV = Dose volume (L/dose)
DT = Dose time (dose/hr)
CFT = Conversion factor time (hr/60 min)
FR = Flow rate in gtt/min
The necessary information needed for using dimensional analysis with this example is as follows:
Drop factor (DF) = 20 gtt/mL
Dose volume (DV) = 1.5 L
Dose time (DT) = 8 hr
FR (flow rate in gtt/min) = x

Conversion Factors 1 L = 1000 mL (CFV); 1 hr = 60 min (CFT)

$$\frac{20 \text{ gtt (DF)}}{1 \text{ mL}} \times \frac{1000 \text{ mL (CFV)}}{1 \text{ L}} \times \frac{1.5 \text{ L (DV)}}{8 \text{ hr}} \times \frac{1 \text{ hr (CFT)}}{60 \text{ min}} = x \text{ gtt/min}$$

$$\frac{20 \text{ gtt}}{1 \text{ mL}} \times \frac{1000 \text{ mL}}{1 \text{ L}} \times \frac{1.5 \text{ L}}{8 \text{ hr}} \times \frac{1 \text{ hr}}{60 \text{ min}} = x$$

$$\frac{20 \text{ gtt} \times 1000 \times 1.5 \times 1}{1 \times 1 \times 8 \times 60} = x$$

$$\frac{30000 \text{ gtt}}{480 \text{ min}} = x$$

$$\frac{3000\cancel{0} \text{ gtt}}{48\cancel{0} \text{ min}} = x$$

$$x = 62.5 \text{ gtt/min or } 63 \text{ gtt/min}$$

If the physician orders a variety of fluids for a given period, such as over 24 hours, the professional should add together all of the fluids for the day and then determine the flow rate, unless the time for infusion varies with each fluid ordered.

When fluids have not infused at the rate expected, whether because the infusion is ahead or behind schedule, determine the amount of fluid remaining in the container and recalculate the flow rate needed to fulfill the physician's order. If this calculation is necessary, the infusion pump or other device that regulates flow rate should be adjusted appropriately. If there is a question of patient safety with the flow rate change, patient safety is the factor that must be considered first. Always check to be sure the change of flow rate will NOT affect how the medication is absorbed if this has a possibility of being a factor. If indicated, contact the physician or pharmacist before changing infusion rates.

CALCULATING IV INFUSION TIMES

In some instances the physician will provide an order for the amount of fluids to be infused and the milliliters per hour without providing the specific running time for the infusion. The problem then is to decide how long it will take for the total infusion using the drop factor ordered by the physician. As the person responsible for the infusion, you have a responsibility to have the container of fluids ordered to follow the current infusion ready when needed. Therefore the time necessary for the current infusion must be calculated. These calculations may be necessary in other circumstances, such as the time needed for completion of the treatment in ambulatory care or for patient discharge or testing following the completion of the infusion.

Basically the formula for determining the time of infusion is the same formula with the unknown being changed.

EXAMPLE USING FORMULA METHOD: A physician orders 1000 mL D-5-S to be administered at 20 gtt/min. The drop factor is 15 gtt/mL. What is the running time (or minutes for infusion) for these fluids?

Using the formula shown in the previous section and substituting information into the formula, the calculation can be made:

$$\text{Flow rate} = \frac{\text{mL ordered} \times \text{gtt/mL (drop factor)}}{\text{min for infusion (Time for infusion)}}$$

$$\text{Flow rate} = 20 \text{ gtt/min}$$
$$\text{mL ordered} = 1000 \text{ mL}$$
$$\text{gtt/mL} = 15 \text{ gtt/mL}$$

With these numbers, the equation will appear as follows:

$$20 \text{ gtt/min} = \frac{1000 \text{ mL} \times 15 \text{ gtt/mL}}{x}$$

$$20 \text{ gtt/min } x = 1000 \text{ mL} \times 15 \text{ gtt/mL}$$
$$20 \text{ gtt/min } x = 1000 \text{ mL} \times 15 \text{ gtt/ mL}$$
$$20 \text{ min } x = 15000$$
$$x = \frac{15000}{20 \text{ min}}$$

$$x = \frac{1500\cancel{0}}{2\cancel{0} \text{ min}}$$

$x = 750$ min or 12.5 hours

(Divide 750 min by 60 min/hour)

EXAMPLE USING DIMENSIONAL ANALYSIS:

A physician orders 1000 mL D-5-S to be administered at 20 gtt/min. The drop factor is 15 gtt/mL. What is the running time for these fluids?

DF = Drop factor

CFV = Conversion factor volume

DV = Dose volume

DT = Dose time

CFT = Conversion factor time

FR = Flow rate in gtt/min

$$DF \times CFV \times DV \times FR = DT$$

Again we will use substitution and complete the equation.

$$DF = 15 \text{ gtt/mL}$$

$$DV = 1000 \text{ mL}$$

$$DT = x$$

$$FR = 20 \text{ gtt/min}$$

$$\frac{15 \text{ gtt (DF)}}{1 \text{ mL}} \times \frac{1000 \text{ mL (CFV)}}{1000 \text{ mL}} \times \frac{1000 \text{ mL (DV)}}{\text{Dose}} \times \frac{\text{Dose}}{20 \text{ gtt/min(FR)}} = DT$$

$$\frac{15 \cancel{\text{gtt}} \text{ (DF)}}{1 \cancel{\text{mL}}} \times \frac{1000 \cancel{\text{mL}} \text{ (CFV)}}{1000 \cancel{\text{mL}}} \times \frac{1000 \cancel{\text{mL}} \text{ (DV)}}{\cancel{\text{Dose}}} \times \frac{\cancel{\text{Dose}}}{20 \cancel{\text{gtt}} /\text{min(FR)}} = DT$$

$$\frac{15 \times 1000 \times 1000}{1 \times 1000 \times 20 \text{min}} = DT$$

$$DT = \frac{15000000}{20000 \text{ min}}$$

$$DT = \frac{1500\cancel{0000}}{2\cancel{0000} \text{ min}}$$

$$DT = \frac{1500}{2} \text{ min}$$

DT=750 min or convert minutes to hours by dividing by 60 minutes/hour = 12.5 hrs.

CALCULATING THE AMOUNT OF A DRUG IN A SOLUTION

Ratio/proportion may be used to determine the amount of medication that is found in a specific amount of solvent. This may require two steps to make the final calculation of the necessary flow rate. The first step will be to determine the number of milliliters of solution needed per time designation to fulfill the physician's order. Then the drops/minute can be determined.

EXAMPLE: A physician orders 5 mg of lorazepam to be added to 500 mL of fluids to be infused at the rate of 1 mg/hr. What is the flow rate in drops per minute that would be correct if using a microdrop infusion set of 15 gtt/mL?

Step 1

$$5 \text{ mg: } 500 \text{ mL:: } 1 \text{ mg: } x$$
$$5 \cancel{\text{mg}}: 500 \text{ mL:: } 1 \cancel{\text{mg}}: x$$
$$5x = 500 \text{ mL}$$
$$x = 100 \text{ mL}$$

Step 2

$$\text{Flow rate} = \frac{\text{mL ordered} \times \text{gtt/mL(drop factor)}}{\text{min for infusion}}$$

$$\text{Flow rate} = \frac{100 \text{ mL} \times 15 \text{ gtt/mL}}{60 \text{ min}}$$

Note that each 100 mL will contain 1 mg of medications and the order is for 1 mg/hr.

$$\text{Flow rate} = \frac{100 \cancel{\text{mL}} \times 15 \text{ gtt/} \cancel{\text{mL}}}{60 \text{ min}}$$

$$\text{Flow rate} = \frac{1500 \text{ gtt}}{60 \text{ min}}$$

$$\text{Flow rate} = 25 \text{ gtt/min}$$

CALCULATING THE AMOUNT OF MEDICATION INFUSED IN THE AMOUNT OF FLUIDS

In some cases the professional who is monitoring an infusion will be required to determine the amount of medication a patient has already received during a certain period of time. To make this determination, use ratio/proportion. The amount of medication in the total solution and the total amount of solution should be placed in one ratio of the proportion and the amount of infused fluids should be placed in the other ratio with "x" being the amount of medication infused.

OR

Total amt of med: Total of fluid:: x (Amt of med infused): Amt of fluid infused

EXAMPLE: A patient receives 750 mL of 1000 mL N/S with 4 mEq KCl added. How many mEq of KCl did the patient receive?

Total amount of medication: Total of fluid:: x (Amount of medication infused): Amount of fluid infused

$$4 \text{ mEq}:1000 \text{ mL}::x:750 \text{ mL}$$

$$4 \text{ mEq}:1000 \text{ mL}::x:750 \text{ mL}$$

$$1000 \, x = 3000 \text{ mEq}$$

$$x = 3000 \text{ mEq}/1000$$

$$x = 3 \text{ mEq}$$

With all calculations for IV infusions, the professional doing the mathematics should be in a quiet place with as few distractions as possible. If the calculation appears to be incorrect or if there is a question about the answer, always ask for assistance. To verify medication amounts that are to be infused, check the orders first and then verify with the pharmacist if appropriate. If the calculation is questionable, recalculate; if there is still a question, ask another professional to check your calculations. Never infuse fluids if there seems to be an error of any kind. Remember that once the fluids have been infused, removal is impossible.

CALCULATING IV MEDICATIONS IN AMOUNTS PER KILOGRAM OF BODY WEIGHT

In some instances the physician may order the amount of medications to be infused per kilogram of body weight over a certain period of time.

The order might read the number of milligrams per kilogram to infuse over a period of time such as minutes.

The first step is to convert the pounds to kilograms using 2.2 pounds per kilogram. The dose of medication for the weight should be calculated. Then convert the weight of the drug to the available medication weight. Finally, the amount of medication per given amount of fluid should be determined using the drop factor of the infusion set.

EXAMPLE: A physician orders ampicillin 5 mg/kg to be infused at 0.25 mg/kg/min for a patient who weighs 154 pounds. The drop factor is 20 gtt/min. What is the total amount of medication that should be administered to the patient? What is the number of milligrams per minute of infusion? What is the time necessary for the infusion?

EXAMPLE USING RATIO/PROPORTION:
Step 1: Convert the pounds to kilograms.

$$154 \text{ \#}: x:: 2.2 \text{ \#}: 1 \text{ kg}$$

$$2.2 \, x = 154 \text{ kg}$$

$$x = 70 \text{ kg}$$

Step 2: Determine the total weight of medication (dose) to be given to the patient.

$$5 \text{ mg/kg}$$

$$\text{Total dose} = 5 \text{ mg} \times 70 \text{ kg}$$

$$\text{Total dose} = 350 \text{ mg}$$

Step 3: Determine the time for administration of the medication by completing the order of the physician for mg/kg/min. The total dose is 350 mg. This medication is to be administered at 0.25 mg/kg/min or 0.25 mg × 70/min or 17.5 mg/min.

Step 4: Determine the administration time in minutes.

$$17.5 \text{ mg}: 1 \text{ min}:: 350 \text{ mg}: x$$

$$17.5 \, x = 350 \text{ min}$$

$$x = 20 \text{ min}$$

EXAMPLE USING FORMULA METHOD:
Using the following formula, calculate the same example.

$$\text{Step 1: } \frac{\text{Dose ordered}}{\text{per kg}} \times \text{total kg} = \text{Dose/min}$$

$$\frac{0.25 \text{ mg}}{1 \text{ kg}} \times 70 \text{ kg} = \text{Dose/min}$$

$$17.5 \text{ mg} = \text{Dose/min}$$

To calculate the time for administration, use the following formula:

$$\text{Step 2: } \frac{\text{Min}}{\text{Dose/min}} \times \text{Total dose} = \text{Time for administration}$$

$$\frac{1 \text{ min}}{17.5 \text{ mg}} \times 350 \text{ mg} = \text{Time for administration}$$

$$\text{Time for administration} = \frac{350 \text{ mg}}{17.5 \text{ mg/min}}$$

$$\text{Time for administration} = 20 \text{ min}$$

REVIEW QUESTIONS

1. A physician orders Kefurox 1.5 G in D-5-S 100 mL to be infiltrated over 1 hour as IVPB (intravenous piggyback). The drop factor is 20 gtt/mL.
   Interpret the order _____
   What is the necessary drip rate (gtt/min) to fulfill this order? _____
   If the patient receives 80 mL of the IVPB, how many milligrams of Kefurox will the patient receive? _____
   If the patient receives the IVPB for 35 minutes, how many mL of solution will the patient receive? _____

2. A physician orders Furosemide 60 mg to be infused in D-5-W 500 mL. The drop factor is 20 gtt/mL and the drip rate is 60 gtt/min. Interpret the order. _____
   How long will the fluids infuse using the drop factor given earlier? _____
   How many milligrams of Furosemide will the patient receive per minute? _____
   What are the total milligrams of Dextrose in the fluids? _____

3. A physician orders Humulin R 60 U added to D-2 1/2-1/2 NS 100 mL as an IVPB. The drop factor is 60 gtt/mL. The physician wants the insulin to infuse at 2.5 U/hr. The label for insulin is Humulin R-100.

Interpret the order _____
How many milliliters per hour will be infused to complete the order? _____
How many milligrams of sodium chloride are found in the fluids? _____
How many milligrams of Dextrose are found in these fluids? _____
How long will the fluids need to infuse as ordered? _____
How many milliliters of insulin will be added to the fluids? _____

4. A physician orders Ampicillin sodium 1 g to be added to Lactated Ringer's 100 mL. The drop factor is 60 gtt/mL. The medication must be given over a 2-hour timeframe.
   Interpret the order. _____
   What will be the flow rate (mL/min) for these fluids? _____
   How many gtt/min will the patient receive? _____
   How many milligrams of medication will be administered in 45 minutes? _____

5. A physician orders Nitro-BID IV 50 mg in D-5-W 250 mL to be infused at the rate of 5 mcg/min. The drop factor is 60 gtt/mL.
   Interpret the order _____
   What is the amount of medication in micrograms per 1 mL of solution? _____
   How many milliliters of solution will be needed to fulfill the order for 50 mcg/mL? ___
   How long will these fluids take to infuse? _____
   How many milliliters will provide Nitro-BID 5 mg? _____

6. A physician orders D-5-S 3000 mL to be infused over 24 hours. The drop factor is 15 gtt/mL.
   Interpret the order. _____
   How many milliliters of fluids should be supplied for each 8-hour shift? _____
   If the fluids are available in 1 L containers, how many containers of solution should be provided for the physician's order? _____
   How many milliliters per hour should be infused? _____
   What is the drip rate in milliliters per minute? _____
   If the physician stops the fluids after 5 hours of infusion, how many milliliters would the patient receive? _____
   How many grams of Dextrose would the patient receive after 5 hours? _____

7. A physician orders Amikin 5 mg/kg/q8h in 100 mL of fluids IVPB. The patient weighs 176 pounds. The drop factor is 20 gtt/mL. The time of infusion is 2 hours.
   How many milligrams of medication should be added to the fluids? ____
   If the medication is available as amikacin 50 mg/mL, how many milliliters should be added to fluids? _____
   What is the flow rate in gtt/min to ensure the medication is given to physician's order? _____

8. What is the time of infusion for D-5-W 1L if the drip rate is 30 mL/min and the drop factor is 20 gtt/mL? _____

   How many bags of fluids would be needed if the physician orders the medications to run for 24 hours? _____

   How many grams of Dextrose will the patient receive with each container of fluids? _____

   How many grams of Dextrose will the patient receive in a 24-hour period? ____

9. A physician orders 500 mL D-5-LR to be infused over 12 hours. The drip factor for the infusion set is 60 gtt/mL. What is the flow rate in mL/min? _____

   How many milliliters of IV fluid will be infused in an hour? _____

10. A physician orders D-2 1/2-1/2 NS 1000 mL for a child who is dehydrated. The physician wants the patient to receive 90 mL the first hour and the remainder over 12 hours. The drop factor is 60 gtt/mL.

    What is the flow rate in millimeters per minute in the first hour? _____

    What is the flow rate in millimeters per minute in the remaining hours? ____

    If the patient only receives 6 hours of fluids, how many mL would the patient receive? _____

    How many grams of Dextrose are in the fluids? _____

    How many grams of sodium chloride are in the fluids? _____

Chapter

6

Foundations of Intravenous Therapy

Chapter Outline

Indications and Rationales for IV Therapy

Methods of Administering IV Medications

Advantages and Disadvantages of IV Therapy

Dangers of IV Therapy

Complications of IV Therapy

Complications after IV Infusion

Evaluating IV Therapy—Its Indications and Risks

Learning Objectives

Upon successful completion of this chapter, the student will be able to:

- List and explain indications for IV therapy.
- Explain the advantages/disadvantages of IV therapy.
- Identify dangers of IV therapy.
- Explain techniques to reduce the complications of IV therapy.
- Discuss infection control and safety related to administration of IV therapy.
- Discuss the risks of IV therapy including localized complications at the

venipuncture/infusion site, systemic/generalized complications, overdose/toxicity, and postinfusion complications.

- Describe the signs and symptoms of local complications and adverse reactions to IV therapy.
- Explain the interventions needed with complications and reactions to IV therapy.

Key Terms

air embolism—presence of air in a blood vessel causing an obstruction.

bolus—concentrated amount of medication given rapidly intravenously.

infiltration—fluid being deposited into tissue.

mechanical problem— physiologic problem that

is created by the mechanics or failure of the mechanics of the procedure.

phlebitis—inflammation of a vein.

pulmonary embolism—presence of an embolism in pulmonary circulation usually resulting in obstruction of blood supply to the pulmonary tissue.

sepsis/septicemia—systemic infection with pathogens present in the circulating blood.

thrombus—clot in the blood vessel; clot is comprised of platelets, fibrin, clotting factors, and blood cells.

The physician's decision to initiate intravenous (IV) therapy involves comparing the indications/rationales for therapy with possible complications that may occur. As with many medical procedures, the immediate and long-term benefits should outweigh any risks involved. This chapter provides information regarding indications/rationale for initiating IV therapy and discusses possible complications as a result of the procedure initiation or continued therapy.

In the ambulatory care setting, IV fluids are administered as intermittent infusions to care for an acute condition that does not require hospitalization. In addition, in an inpatient setting, IV fluids also are given to maintain fluid intakes during illness, reestablish plasma volume, replace electrolyte losses resulting from gastrointestinal diseases, and provide nutrition in patients who cannot consume sufficient calories daily to maintain homeostasis.

INDICATIONS AND RATIONALES FOR IV THERAPY

The indications or rationales for using IV therapy fall into three categories: maintenance therapy, replacement therapy, and restoration therapy. Additional indications for initiating and maintaining restoration IV therapy include the establishment of access to a vein for administration of medications and fluids required to maintain fluid, electrolyte balance, or both and for administration of medications that cannot be ingested by oral route. IVs also provide a ready-available access for treatment by keeping the vein open. An IV that is administered at a very slow rate to maintain access to the vein is often referred to as keep open (KO) so it is available for immediate access for emergency situations or for administration of medications. This is important because it refers to the ability to have a route for medication administration when rapid response is required. Further indications include administration of blood and blood components, administration of chemotherapy, administration of anesthesia or diagnostic reagents, and administration of medication using a **bolus** or piggyback setup. IV administration of drugs and fluids is useful in patients who are unconscious or are unable to ingest food.

Maintenance therapy involves providing necessary nutrients for daily needs of water, electrolytes, and nutrition for the patients having reduced or no intake of oral fluids and nutritional elements. IV infusions provide a method for the health care provider to maintain hydration in the patient with dehydration from gastrointestinal disorders, such as diarrhea, and in those who cannot take fluids by the oral route. The maintenance of fluid balance is essential to maintain the body's state of equilibrium.

Replacement therapy is indicated when the patient has experienced a deficit in the intake of fluids and nourishment, usually over a period of 48 hours or more. As previously mentioned in Chapter 2, a large part of the body's fluid is water that is divided into two main compartments: intracellular and extracellular. To assist the body in the maintenance of homeostasis and fluid balance, IV fluids and electrolytes are administered.

The amount of water in the body is a response to fluid intake and fluid output. Normally, an average-size adult will have a daily intake of approximately 3000 mL of fluid. Many factors influence the normal intake of fluids, including the intake of liquids, the consumption of food, and the oxidization of nutrients during metabolism. Fluid output is normally about the same amount as the intake. Normally, body fluids are lost in urine, feces, perspiration, and respiration. Vomiting, diarrhea, hemorrhage, profuse sweating, and exposure to excessive heat may cause excessive fluid loss and consequent dehydration. During these processes, electrolytes also are depleted. When disease conditions and emergent situations are responsible for extensive fluid loss, fluid replacement must be accomplished by alternative means, usually IV infusion.

Restorative therapy involves daily restoration of fluids and electrolytes. Laboratory testing is necessary to determine the amount of electrolytes and fluids lost and what is required to replace them on a daily basis. Therefore, this therapy is most often performed in an inpatient setting.

In the event that medication cannot be administered orally, because of the inability to swallow the medication, the detremental effects of the gastrointestinal secretions, or the drugs, the IV infusion or injection becomes an essential route for the drug therapy. For any medication, including electrolytes, to be effective, it must reach the blood for distribution throughout the body. Oral medications are absorbed through the digestive tract, and parenteral medications other than those given intravenously cross tissue barriers before absorption. With IV therapy, these barriers do not exist and the entire amount of medication is distributed in the bloodstream immediately after administration. Thus, one of the major indications and advantages of IV therapy is the rapid absorption of medication, but this too could become a major disadvantage when errors or adverse reactions occur.

Certain drugs cannot be administered orally or by other routes. Contents of the gastrointestinal (GI) tract often interact with oral medications, rendering them less effective or useless. Others cannot be absorbed in the GI tract. Some patients are unable to take medications by mouth because of an inability to swallow or level of consciousness. Others may be vomiting or may be uncooperative and thus unable to have oral medications administered. IV therapy becomes an important asset for the health care provider and the patient to provide drugs in emergency situations and when rapid absorption of a medication is needed.

Common medications that are administered intravenously include antimicrobial agents such as cephalosporins, aminoglycosides, and penicillins. Other classifications of drugs that may be administered by the IV route include anticoagulants, antifungals, antiviral agents, bronchodilators, hypoglycemic drugs, insulin, immunosuppressants, biotherapy drugs, and neuromuscular blocking agents. Chemotherapy drugs may also be administered by IV therapy, usually as an infusion. Opioid drugs may be delivered in a bolus form for intermittent pain relief or continuous analgesia. Refer to Chapter 7 for more information about IV medication.

METHODS OF ADMINISTERING IV MEDICATIONS

IV therapy involves the administration of medications or drug therapy using the following methods: continuous infusion, either as intermittent infusion, bolus injection, or piggyback infusion. IV fluids themselves are considered a type of drug therapy in the form of isotonic, hypotonic, or hypertonic solutions. Additionally, chemical replacements such as electrolytes may be added to the solution to manage homeostasis and fluid balance. Medications such as bronchodilators or a hypoglycemic agent (insulin) may be added for administration at a controlled and slow drip rate. Narcotics used for pain relief may be added to the fluids for patient-controlled analgesia with the patient dispensing anesthesia as needed for pain relief.

Controlled drip rates, as ordered by the physician, must be maintained when medications are added to the primary bag of solution. This is a necessary action to prevent an overdose of the medication. Methods of controlling the drip rate are discussed in Chapter 4 under the discussion of equipment.

Bolus injections may be administered through an existing IV line or directly into a vein. Bolus injections are often drawn up in a syringe and administered through an access port by way of slow or rapid push. When giving the bolus into an existing IV line, the health care provider inserts the medication-filled syringe into the access port and pushes the plunger of the syringe at the prescribed rate. If a bolus injection is introduced directly into a vein, care should be taken to dilute the medications as indicated and provide at a rate necessary for patient safety. **CAUTION:** This type of IV medication administration is beyond the scope of an untrained health care professional. Physicians, paramedics, specially trained registered nurses, and radiology technicians are the health care professionals who administer drugs by the IV bolus push route. Refer to practice acts and legislation of your state and community and to facility guidelines found in the policy manual for information on administration by bolus push.

IV piggyback (IVPB) is a secondary set that is attached to the primary administration set. As previously mentioned, medications dissolved in the smaller amount of solution can be administered using this route without disconnecting the primary IV line. This type of administration is often used for dosages to be administered at regular intermittent intervals (i.e., every 8 hours). Different from IV bolus, IVPB provides medications that have been diluted but the ordered flow rate for the fluids must be carefully followed. Refer to Chapter 4 for additional information.

ADVANTAGES AND DISADVANTAGES OF IV THERAPY

Although IV therapy is often a necessary intervention in the treatment of a patient, the procedure carries some risk even when all precautions are taken and no break in sterile or medical aseptic techniques occur. The health care professional must be alert of possible complications at all stages of IV therapy. The inherent dangers and the methods that can reduce the complications of IV therapy are discussed as complications of IV therapy to follow. Individuals who are dehydrated; vomiting; experiencing electrolyte imbalance; unconscious; in shock; or unable to take medications, fluids, or nourishment orally benefit from IV therapy as fluids and electrolytes are replaced. The more rapid absorption of antibiotics and other medications is another advantage. Many antibiotics require specific blood levels to be maintained to reach optimum benefits. Other medications also often require that blood levels remain constant to be effective. Because of many factors, oral intake is not always the route that will achieve the constant levels required for maximum benefit to the patient.

DANGERS OF IV THERAPY

Most dangers are associated with human error, whereas complications are from the IV fluids. An obvious danger of IV therapy is the possible introduction of microorganisms directly into the bloodstream when aseptic technique is not followed precisely. Because fluids are introduced directly into the bloodstream for transport throughout the body, the strictest of aseptic techniques is necessary. Any possible loss of asepsis must be confronted and the equipment must be discarded to protect the patient. Remember sterility is not measured in degrees. Please refer to Chapter 3 on asepsis for additional information on the prevention of sepsis and the importance of sterile technique.

Other dangers include safety issues related to human errors that are associated with the medication calculations. Chapter 5 addresses the importance of calculating the correct dosage of medication for infusion. Review of basic concepts of infection control; correct dosage; and calculations, including of weight and volume of the metric system, are necessary for patient safety and the prevention of dangerous conditions. Information including the importance of the correct flow rate ensures that fluids are administered during the specific prescribed time. The use of the seven rights and three befores helps to ensure that the patient is receiving the correct medication, the danger to the patient is reduced, and patient safety is reinforced.

The health care professional has the responsibility of continually observing the infusion site and the patient's general status to detect any complications that may arise and caring for these complications in a timely manner to prevent further insult. Patient safety must always be of primary importance. A discussion of complications and risks of IV therapy follows.

COMPLICATIONS OF IV THERAPY

Complications of IV therapy can be of different origins. They may be local at the infusion site or generalized and systemic. Local complications include **mechanical problems** such as **infiltration** into the surrounding tissue, a leak of fluid at the site, or a displaced catheter. Localized infection within the vein or **phlebitis** can result from a break in asepsis. Systemic complications include circulatory overload, phlebitis, **thrombus** formation, **pulmonary embolism, air embolism,** or generalized infection. The possibility of drug overdose and toxicity exists with the introduction of medication directly into the bloodstream. Because of the many chances of complications and possible dangers of IV therapy, careful monitoring of patients receiving medication is crucial. After the infusion is discontinued, possible complications may include bleeding at the site—excessive bleeding or even hemorrhaging—that demands prompt management. Mechanical problems related to the infusion system or trauma to the veins may be the causes of delayed local adverse reactions.

Local Complications

Local complications may occur at the initiation of the IV, during the IV infusion, and after the IV catheter or needle is removed. Some of the problems include infiltration of fluids into the surrounding tissues caused by improper placement of the needle, trauma to the vein on insertion of the needle, or leaving the tourniquet in place following the initiation of the flow of fluids.

Infiltration
Description of Complication
Infiltration of fluids into the surrounding tissues occurs when the device used for insertion of the IV line is displaced from the vein, or fluid leaks from the vein, allowing the fluid to flow into the tissue.

Symptoms and Signs
The patient may be the first person to realize that difficulty is occurring because the skin will feel tight and appear stretched and taut, with increasing discomfort at the infusion site. The signs are usually seen close to the insertion site including slowing or stopping of the fluid infusion, tissue induration, and swelling around the injection site with tissue remaining cool to touch. With the use of infusion devices, the chance of continued infiltration is less likely to occur because an alarm sounds when the fluids infiltrate.

Treatment
Lowering of the IV bag below the venipuncture site provides a process for a quick check to determine if the IV has infiltrated. If there is a blood return, the IV is still in the vein. When no blood return is evident, the device for the IV apparently has been displaced from the vein.

When this complication occurs, the IV is discontinued and the needle or catheter for infusion is removed. The infusion site will have to be changed and the affected limb will need to be elevated and covered with warm compresses or other therapy as ordered by the physician or as directed by the local policies. Observations and actions should be documented, and the IV infusion should be restarted at another site. When a small amount of fluid remains to be infused, the physician should be contacted to see if a restart is necessary. The health care professional has the responsibility of caring for these complications in a timely manner to prevent further trauma to the tissues. As a means of decreasing tissue damage, the IV site should be observed every hour and the tubing should be secured in a manner as to prevent movement of the tubing and the hub of the cannula.

Hematomas and Ecchymosis
Description
Hematomas and ecchymosis may be found when a tourniquet is placed above the infusion site, the vein is nicked, or a leaky vein occurs because of frequent use of the same vein for venipuncture or IV therapy. When a venipuncture site used is distal to a previous site, leakage may occur from that site. Blood seeps or leaks into the tissue, causing the pooling of blood and forming the hematoma or the area of bruising. The use of the most distal possible vein in initiating the IV helps to prevent this complication. This complication is preventable with careful venipuncture technique and the correct placement of the tourniquet.

Symptoms and Signs
Discoloration of the skin, swelling, and discomfort are the most frequent signs. The health care professional has the responsibility to inspect the

infusion site for these complications on a regular, systematic basis. Just because the patient does not complain does not mean that regular care for the site should not take place.

Treatment

Assess the situation, and usually the cannula or needle will need to be removed. Elevate the affected limb and apply warm compresses. The remaining fluid amount is assessed and when sufficient quantity remains, the IV is restarted. Should only a small amount of fluid remain to be infused, contact the physician for orders to discontinue or restart. Assessment and interventions must be documented.

Leakage of Fluid Around the Venipuncture Site
Description of Complication

Leakage of fluid around the venipuncture site creates another dilemma. IV fluid leaks around the infusion device or from the connection of the device to the IV tubing. In addition, bleeding from the venipuncture site may occur during the infusion.

Symptoms and Signs

Often times the cannula or needle has become slightly dislodged, allowing for the fluid to run out of the site onto the dressing. The patient complains that the dressing covering the insertion site feels wet and cool. This circumstance sets up an excellent medium for pathogens to establish residence in the dressing. Observation of the amount of fluid infused indicating that the infusion is ahead of schedule may signify that fluid is leaking out around the venipuncture site. As a result of this complication, the quantity of IV fluid and medication entering the circulatory system is diminished and the patient may not receive the amount of medication ordered.

Treatment

The dressing should be removed and the cannula should be checked to see that it is still in the vein at the proper distance; if it is not, attempts are made to reposition it to the proper distance. When

it is not possible to reposition the cannula, then the cannula is removed and a sterile dressing is applied to the site. The connection of the insertion device and the tubing should be checked to ensure that it has not come loose, permitting fluid to leak out from the tubing prior to reaching the vein. When the fluid is actually leaking around the cannula or needle and readjustment of the insertion device does not correct the problem, the device is removed and a sterile dressing is applied to the site. A new site is located and the IV is restarted with new sterile equipment.

When leakage is the result of a poor connection, the IV is discontinued and restarted with new equipment because the tubing connection and the hub of the cannula are now considered to be contaminated.

Infection

Infection from IV therapy can be localized or generalized throughout the body through the bloodstream. The first line of defense of protecting the patient from infection as a result of IV therapy is the practice of good and consistent handwashing, proper medical asepsis, and maintenance of sterility as appropriate. A number of infections are nosocomial in origin. The health care professional must be assured that CDC standards are followed before there is contact with any IV equipment, solutions, or medications. Additionally, other potential sources of IV-related causes of contamination, including problems during manufacturing, packaging, or storage, should be evaluated prior to fluid use. Blood remaining in the tubing when blood is allowed to flow back into the tubing postvenipuncture may be another possible source of infection. Another source could be a break in aseptic technique during the therapy. Injection ports must be properly cleansed with an aseptic solution prior to the administration of any medication or solution. All needles and devices used to insert medication or solutions into ports must be sterile, and the added medications or fluids should be prepared in a manner that preserves sterility as appropriate.

Localized Infections at the Venipuncture Site

Description

The practice of medical asepsis and sterile technique when starting the IV is the first step in preventing an infection at the venipuncture site. The breach in the integrity of the skin with the venipuncture disturbs the body's first line of defense against the invasion of pathogens. Proper cleansing of the intended site before the venipuncture and the application of a sterile dressing to the site postpuncture are proactive measures for limiting the incidence of infection, as is the importance of maintaining sterility of IV equipment that will be introduced to the vein.

Symptoms and Signs

Symptoms and signs of an infection include swelling, redness, and pain in the area. A purulent discharge also may be present at the site. The skin in the surrounding area usually is warmer than normal. Red streaks may radiate from the site or area and the patient may experience a fever and chills. The white blood cell count often is elevated.

Treatment

The usual course of action is to discontinue the IV and remove the catheter or needle to study it for culture and sensitivity. Antiseptic ointment may be applied and a new sterile dressing should be placed over the site. Observations and actions are charted. A new site is selected and the IV is restarted usually with new tubing and needle or infusion device if it is determined that the fluids have not been compromised, or according to the policies of the facility. It is common practice to inspect and change the dressing every 24 hours, which is important in preventing local infections. Additionally, if the patient complains of pain in the area, the site should be checked for any indication of infection or infiltration. Remember, good aseptic technique is essential in preventing any infectious process.

Systemic Complications

Systemic complications include **sepsis/septicemia;** circulatory overload; and vascular complications such as phlebitis, thrombus, and embolus (pulmonary and air embolus). Overdose, toxicity, or both also may occur when too much of a medication is infused, the medication is infused too rapidly, or the dosage is not calculated correctly. (Refer to Chapter 5 for methods for calculating in safe IV therapy.) The health care professional responsible for overseeing the IV therapy must be alert to any change in the patient's condition indicative of the early onset of a systemic complication. Once a systemic problem is suspected, immediate intervention is mandated to prevent life-threatening complications.

Sepsis/Septicemia

Description

Generalized infection or sepsis may occur when pathogens enter the blood through the IV fluids or from pathogens present on the tubing that are able to migrate from the equipment through the venipuncture into the blood. Another source may be the IV fluids themselves that are contaminated, thus introducing pathogens into the body.

Symptoms and Signs

The patient will exhibit signs and symptoms of generalized infection including chills and fever, increasing heart and respiratory rate, and dropping blood pressure. The white blood count is usually elevated. He or she may display anxiety and restlessness or lethargy, and complain of not feeling "right" or will say "Something is wrong." This may be a delayed reaction after the IV has been discontinued. Any reports of these signs and symptoms, either during or after infusion, should be taken seriously and reported to the physician immediately.

Treatment

In most cases, after blood cultures have been obtained, the physician will order appropriate antibiotics to be administered. An open IV line is necessary for maintenance of fluid intake. Vital signs are monitored and recorded on a regular basis. The patient must be carefully watched for possible life-threatening situations.

Fluid Overload

When IV fluids are infused too rapidly, systemic complications such as cardiac overload and respiratory difficulties may occur. All infusion rates should be responsibly checked at least twice prior to administration, even if the rate has been calculated by another health care professional. Remember that the person performing the infusion is responsible for his or her actions, including the calculation of the flow rate. Checking the infusion rate on a regular basis after the infusion has started also is a responsibility that cannot be denied. Each time the patient is checked, the flow rates should also be checked by the responsible health care professional. Any shortness of breath or swelling should be followed closely, vital signs should be obtained, and the physician should be notified of the patient's condition on a regular basis if the early signs of complications are observed.

Circulatory Overload
Description

Circulatory overload is a major complication that can be life threatening if prompt intervention does not occur. An infusion administered too rapidly or reduced kidney function may be responsible for this major complication. Impaired cardiac contraction as a result of increased blood volume does not allow for adequate blood supply to reach the kidneys for filtration and excretion.

Symptoms and Signs

In the early stages of fluid overload, the patient will display apprehension and some shortness of breath. Pulse, respiratory rates, and blood pressure

increase. As the amount of the overload increases, the patient may exhibit additional shortness of breath, anxiety, elevated blood pressure, and a bounding pulse. Both respirations and pulse become more rapid. Edema is often present around the eyes and in the limbs, especially hands and ankles. Neck and limb veins appear distended. Skin appears taut and shiny, and there may be peripheral cyanosis. Capillary refill is delayed. Fluid is auscultated in the lungs. If possible to weigh the patient, a weight gain from before the onset of therapy is usually noted. Congestive heart failure and pulmonary edema are sequelae that may be seen.

Treatment

The IV flow rate should be slowed and the physician should be contacted. If available, provide the patient with oxygen and assist into a semi-Fowler's position. Vital signs should be taken and recorded. All observations and interventions should be documented. The usual course of treatment ordered by the physician includes slowing the infusion rate and administering diuretics to remove excess fluid from the body. Intake and output are carefully monitored with desired urinary output being in excess of 60 mL/hr.

Remember, calculations of flow rates should be checked at least twice before the infusion begins and then at least every hour during the infusion. Controllers or infusion devices should be used in patients at greatest risk for complications. Time-tapes applied to the fluid container indicate the amount of fluid that should be administered each hour. These tapes provide an easy indication of whether the fluids are infusing too rapidly or too slowly.

Vascular Complications
Phlebitis
Description

Phlebitis, an inflammatory process in the vein, may occur above the infusion site if the therapy is given on successive days, or with an irritating substance being administered through the vein.

Symptoms and Signs

Phlebitis is indicated by at least two of the following signs: redness, pain, swelling, or warmth at the site. Red streaks may radiate from the site. Pain and tenderness are noted in the affected area along the vein. The inflammation may cause the vein to feel like a cord. The vein should be assessed regularly for this sign, especially if the IV therapy occurs over a prolonged period.

Treatment

The IV is discontinued and restarted at another site. Warm compresses may be applied to the area, and observations and actions should be documented.

Thrombus
Description

The formation of a thrombus, a blood clot that obstructs a blood vessel, often is the result of stasis of blood at the catheter or needle tip or in the vein.

Symptoms and Signs

Indications of this condition include a slowing infusion rate, swelling, and discomfort. Often, the thrombus can be felt as a firm, threadlike formation along the course of the vein.

Treatment

The IV is discontinued, a sterile dressing is applied to the infusion site, and the IV is restarted at another site (preferably in the other limb). The physician is notified and warm compresses may be applied to the site. Again, observations and actions are documented. The physician may order thrombolytics to assist with dissolving the thrombus.

Embolus
Description

An embolus is a clot of aggregated material, such as bits of tumor tissue cells, air bubbles, bacteria, or foreign bodies. The embolus can lodge in any vessel and inhibit the blood flow beyond the obstruction.

Symptoms and Signs

The symptoms of an embolus depend on the location of the occluded vessel and the magnitude of the area of the tissue served by the vessel. Initial symptoms include severe pain in the area of the embolus. Emboli lodging in arteries of the extremities cause the area to become pale, numb, and cold to touch. Emboli consequential to IV therapy usually are in the veins, with the most severe area of involvement being the pulmonary vessels. Pulmonary embolism is discussed in the following text.

Treatment

Treatment of an embolism in a limb is to elevate the limb and to immobilize it to prevent movement. The physician is notified and specific symptomatic treatment is instituted. All observations and interventions are documented.

Pulmonary Embolism
Description

A pulmonary embolism occurs when a mass of foreign material lodges in and occludes an artery in the pulmonary circulation resulting in the interruption of blood supply to the area. This is caused by the migration of a clot from the limb to the pulmonary circulation, where it becomes lodged in a smaller pulmonary vessel. A pulmonary embolism is one of the most severe complications, and support with ventilation is necessary.

Symptoms and Signs

Symptoms and signs are determined by the size and location of the embolism along with the general physical condition of the patient. Apprehension is common in these patients at the onset of the obstruction and during the course of treatment. The patient with a small, uncomplicated embolism experiences a cough, chest pain, and low-grade fever. The patient with more extensive infarction will experience sudden onset of chest pain, acute shortness of breath, dyspnea, and tachypnea with extreme anxiety. The heart rate will become very rapid and blood pressure drops significantly.

Treatment

This life-threatening occurrence demands immediate intervention. The physician is notified immediately and oxygen is administered. Physician presence to manage the emergency is required. Anticoagulant medications (usually heparin) are ordered and administered. When applicable, thrombolytic drugs may be administered to dissolve the clot. Without immediate aggressive intervention, a pulmonary embolism rapidly may become fatal.

Air Embolism

Description

Similar to a pulmonary embolism, an air embolism occurs when a large air bubble enters the systemic circulation and is transported to the pulmonary circulation. The air mass causes an interruption in blood flow in the pulmonary vessels.

Symptoms and Signs

The individual experiencing an air embolism will display signs and symptoms similar to those of a pulmonary embolism. This potentially lethal condition demands the same immediate intervention as described for pulmonary embolism. This situation occurs when large air bubbles enter the circulatory system often as the result of large air bubbles not being purged from the IV tubing prior to the fluid administration. Care must be taken at all times to ensure that air is not in the tubing and therefore not infused into the circulation with the IV fluids.

Treatment

Treatment is similar to that of pulmonary embolism. Oxygen is administered to the patient. Vital signs are monitored and the physician is notified. All observations and interventions must be documented.

Overdose/Toxicity

Description

Medications used to treat respiratory conditions (theophylline), hyperglycemia (insulin), cardiac arrhythmias (lidocaine), hypotension (dopamine), or hypertension (hydralazine [Apresoline]) may cause an overdose or toxicity when an excess dose of medication is infused. Drug overdose or toxicity may be caused by any medication administered by IV route, not only the commonly used drugs. Drug blood levels must be monitored frequently and the patient must be observed closely. The drugs have a very small margin of error in dosage; therefore the patient receiving these medications by IV continuous infusion or bolus is at risk for overdose and resulting toxicity. The previously listed drugs are only a portion of medications that may be administered during IV therapy. Refer to Chapter 7 for a review of drugs administered by IV route.

Symptoms and Signs

Because any drug that is administered during IV therapy may cause toxicity, any unusual symptoms occurring during the administration must be considered to be serious. Any symptoms detected should be recorded and brought to the attention of the physician.

Symptoms and signs vary according to the drug level and the drug that is causing the symptoms. The patient who is theophylline toxic will exhibit signs of overstimulation of the central nervous system, including nervousness, restlessness, tremors, and possibly convulsions. Additionally they may have gastric upset and tachycardia. The patient experiencing insulin overdose may exhibit the signs of insulin reaction, including anxiety, tachycardia, irritability, trembling, cool moist skin with perspiration, confusion, seizures, and loss of consciousness. Lidocaine is often given by bolus or by continuous drip. Patients with toxemia often exhibit signs of GI distress, lightheadedness, and tremors. Dopamine is used in an emergent or possible maintenance situation to treat hypotension. Toxicity will be demonstrated by a hypertensive reaction. When the patient with hypertension being treated with Apresoline or any other antihypertensive IV medication becomes toxic, the primary symptom will be a sudden or gradual hypotensive state.

Treatment

Treatment involves slowing or discontinuing the IV drip or medication, assessing vital signs, notifying the physician, documenting observation and events, and continuing to monitor the patient and the situation. When an antidote is indicated, the physician will order it. The patient should not be left alone until he or she is stabilized.

COMPLICATIONS AFTER IV INFUSION

After the infusion is discontinued, complications, including bleeding at the site or hemorrhaging, can occur and these demand prompt management. Mechanical problems related to the infusion system or trauma to the veins may be the causes of delayed local adverse reactions.

Bleeding Following IV Therapy
Description

Bleeding at the previous venipuncture site may occur once the cannula has been removed. The bleeding may occur immediately or the onset may be delayed if the blood clot is dislodged.

Symptoms and Signs

Bleeding occurs as the cannula is removed and it may not be controlled by gentle pressure. As the bleeding continues and is not controlled by conventional methods, the patient may become apprehensive. Usually a pressure dressing halts the blood flow in a short time. However, delayed bleeding may occur after a dressing has been applied to the venipuncture site.

The patient will complain of the hand feeling damp or wet and cold. Inspection reveals the presence of blood flow that has not been controlled by the dressing. The dressing usually is saturated, and clothing, blankets, sheets, or drapes may have blood on them.

Treatment

Treatment involves controlling the bleeding. Gentle pressure is applied and the dressing is not removed but reinforced with a pressure dressing. Vital signs are monitored and reassurance is provided. If the bleeding subsides but oozing is still present, the outline of the blood saturation and the time of the outline is marked on the dressing. If the bleeding continues and efforts to control it are not successful, the physician should be notified and all assessments and interventions should be documented. Additional pressure dressings are to be applied over the previous dressing until the physician can assess the situation.

EVALUATING IV THERAPY—ITS INDICATIONS AND RISKS

The comparison of indications for and risks of IV therapy are considered before the decision to initiate IV therapy is made. The immediate and long-term benefits should outweigh any risks involved. IV fluids are administered to maintain fluid intake during illnesses, to reestablish plasma volume, to replace electrolyte losses resulting from gastrointestinal diseases, and to provide nutrition in patients who cannot consume sufficient calories daily. Additional indications for IV therapy include the establishment of access to a vein for administration of medications or fluids required to maintain fluid or electrolyte balance and the establishment of a route to administer medications that cannot be ingested orally. Keeping an open vein for treatment or treatment intervention is used to maintain availability for immediate access. This provides a route for medication administration when rapid response is required. Further indications include administration of blood and blood components, administration of chemotherapy, administration of anesthesia or diagnostic reagents, and administration of medication using a bolus or piggyback (IVPB) setup. IV administration of drugs and fluids is useful in patients who are unconscious.

IV therapy is not without risks. The physician has weighed the benefits against the risks and has made the decision to initiate the therapy.

The health care professional who initiates, maintains, and terminates the therapy has a responsibility to the patient to be alert at all stages of IV therapy to possible complications and to provide prompt intervention if necessary. The health care professional also has the responsibility to use aseptic technique and follow all aseptic precautions to prevent the possibility of infection. The health care provider must be alert at all stages of the IV therapy for any untoward effect of the therapy and ready to provide immediate and proper intervention.

REVIEW QUESTIONS

1. List the three categories of rationales or indications for IV therapy.
2. What factors influence the normal intake of fluids?
3. What are some of the drugs that may be administered by IV route?
4. List methods for the administration of IV medications.
5. What type of patient benefits from IV therapy?
6. What are the symptoms and signs of infiltration?
7. What is the first line of defense to prevent infection?
8. Describe the symptoms and signs of sepsis/septicemia.
9. Describe the symptoms and signs of circulatory overload.
10. Describe the symptoms and signs of pulmonary embolism.

Chapter 7

Pharmacology Related to Intravenous Therapy

Chapter Outline

Principles of Safe Administration of Medications

Patient Assessment Needs Related to Medications

Pharmacokinetics Related to IV Therapy

IV Pharmacology Related to Body Systems

Total Parenteral Nutrition

Incompatibilities of Fluids and Medications

Safety Considerations

Learning Objectives

Upon successful completion of this chapter, the student will be able to:

- Provide an understanding of the essential importance of using the seven rights and three befores in administering IV medications.
- Provide the needed information that will assist in ensuring that quality patient safety is provided during IV therapy.
- Ensure that the pharmacokinetics (absorption, distribution, metabolism, and excretion) of medications in general and the rapidity of these processes with IV infusions are understood.

- Review basic drugs used for IV therapy by drug classification and the body system that is most frequently affected.
- Furnish the basic information of drug compatibilities and incompatibilities including listing those medications that are incompatible with basic IV fluids.
- Convey the basic information to provide patient safety during the administration of medications using IV infusion.

Key Terms

absorption—uptake of medications into the body through or across tissues.

agonist—medication that binds to the receptor site and stimulates the function of that site; a drug that mimics a function of the body.

antagonist—medication that binds to the receptor site to prevent other medications

from binding to those sites; cancellation or reduction of one drug's effect by another drug.

bactericidal—pertaining to the destruction of bacteria; drugs or chemicals that can destroy bacteria.

bacteriostatic—inhibiting or retarding growth of bacteria; drugs or chemicals that can

inhibit or retard growth of bacteria.

continuous infusion—an uninterrupted injection of a liquid substance into the vein.

distribution—dispersion of medication particles to sites in the body.

excretion—elimination of a medication from the body.

extravasate—to escape from the vessel into the tissue.

idiosyncratic reaction—unexpected, unusual response to a drug.

intermittent infusion—administration of medications or an infusion that is not continuous but is interrupted between doses.

IV injection (IV push)—the use of a needle attached to a syringe to instill a single dose of medication into a vein.

metabolism—physical or chemical processes in the body that inactivate a drug for excretion; biotransformation.

narcotic—older term for a controlled drug that depresses the central nervous system to relieve pain and has the potential to cause habituation or addiction.

opiate—drug containing or derived from opium.

opioid—drug that is a synthetic analgesic with the strength of a morphine-like substance but is not derived from opium.

patient controlled analgesia (PCA)—a controlled infusion that allows the patient to administer a predetermined amount of analgesic.

peripheral parenteral nutrition (PPN)—method of administering diluted nutritional substances in a peripheral IV site.

pharmacokinetics—processing of drugs in the body.

superinfection—new infection that appears during the course of treatment for a primary infection.

total parenteral nutrition (TPN)—providing nutritional support through a central IV route.

As with all administration of medications, the professional responsible for the intravenous infusion also has many responsibilities other than just starting the infusion. As discussed in Chapter 5, the calculation of the accurate dose and dosage is most important because medications that have been given intravenously cannot be retrieved. The patient assessment prior to infusion is important so that any changes in the patient's condition can be evaluated based on correct and current information. The importance of understanding the pharmacology of a medication prior to administration cannot be stressed enough.

Legally it is the responsibility of the person administering the medication to be aware of the dosage, indications, side effects, adverse reactions, and allergic reactions to any medication being given. This text cannot cover each medication and its potential problems; therefore the professional should always use reference materials prior to giving drugs, being sure the information is correct as understood. The reference materials should be readily accessible, and this responsibility, both legally and ethically, cannot be overlooked. The professional should have the accurate knowledge base to protect the patient by knowing the physician's order for the IV fluids is complete, correct, and appropriate for the patient's physical condition.

PRINCIPLES OF SAFE ADMINISTRATION OF MEDICATIONS

Early in any medical professional career in which the responsibility for administering medications will be used, the seven rights and three befores are taught. Recall that medication labels should be read *before* taking from storage, *before* pouring, and *before* returning the medication to the storage site. The seven *rights* of medication administration are also necessary:

• Right Drug
• Right Dose
• Right Time
• Right Route
• Right Patient
• Right Technique
• Right Documentation

By following these rules and having knowledge of the medication being infused, patient safety is enhanced and better ensured. These steps are important also in reducing the chance for legal considerations later.

PATIENT ASSESSMENT NEEDS RELATED TO MEDICATIONS

As a review of patient differences to medication, the professional should assess the patient for allergies to foods, drugs, and environmental factors. Sensitivities in one area may be transferred when medications are given. Another necessary area of assessment is the lifestyle of the patient and the availability of resources for care, as appropriate. This could include the actual care that is available or it could be the knowledge level of the patient and the ability of the person who will be caregiver to understand the needed care. In some cases, this may present a problem in ensuring the regimen of the physician is followed. Finally, any area that may alter the response to the medication should be evaluated, including genetic factors, preexisting conditions or illnesses, and age. Age, genetics, amount of body fat, and preexisting conditions of body organs that influence absorption, distribution, metabolism, or excretion of administered drugs will also influence the manner in which the patient responds to the treatment.

Even when the evaluation of the patient produces some expected possible problems with IV infusion, the danger comes from the unexpected and undesired effects that may occur. These reactions are not side effects because side effects, although undesirable, are not completely unexpected. Rather, these unexpected effects can be life-threatening, including such responses as drug allergies, tolerance to medication over a period of time, an accumulation of medication because of the composition of the body tissues, or an **idiosyncratic reaction.** The unpredictable idiosyncrasy, such as the person who is stimulated by diphenhydramine (Benadryl) rather than sedated, does not cause hypersensitivity or allergies but may cause detrimental effects for the patient. The unwanted reactions may also be beneficial when the drug has been given to provide a certain response, such as cyproheptadine (Periactin)

being used for patients who need to gain weight. Therefore the patient must be assessed early on and must be carefully followed throughout the entire infusion and for a time thereafter.

Again, this section is only a review of information that has been presented in other chapters of this text. This cannot be reiterated too many times, however, because of the need to protect patient safety and to reduce the opportunities for legal actions. The health care professional must always be cognizant of the patient and the need for safe medical care.

PHARMACOKINETICS RELATED TO IV THERAPY

Pharmacokinetics, from the terms *pharmaco-* meaning drugs and *-kinesis* for movement, relates to how the body processes medications, including the IV fluids, and is the base for the administration of the medications. The four processes of pharmacokinetics include **absorption, distribution, metabolism** or transformation, and **excretion.** First, with IV administration of medications, the absorption rate is immediate because the drug is injected directly into the bloodstream and absorption through other organs into the bloodstream is not necessary.

Second, the distribution of the drug is not slowed because of the rate of absorption. One of the major dangers of IV medication administration is the immediate distribution throughout the body because the medication is injected immediately in the bloodstream. Although the drug is delivered to the organ or tissues through blood vessels and capillaries, the effect is on the tissues, not on the blood vessels. The amount of drug circulating in the blood is called the drug blood level, and with IV drugs, this is the amount that is infused. At the site for the body's use of the drug, barriers such as blood–brain membrane barriers and cell permeability may slow the absorption at the distribution site, but the time is not as slow as would be found with other routes of administration that must be disintegrated and absorbed into the bloodstream.

The site of use for the medication will remain as found with the oral or other parenteral forms of the medication. Medications are chosen to be effective for certain conditions at specific physical sites. The selectivity of medications to certain body cells allows some treatment to specific body cells and organs, such as thyroid replacements, whereas other drugs, such as antibiotics, are less selective and are distributed to multiple types of cells throughout the body.

After the drug reaches its site of distribution, a series of chemical reactions occur—converting the medication to be broken down for use, and then prepared for the body to rid itself of the medication that has not been utilized. The primary site for metabolism is the liver so any liver condition would affect the amount of medication the patient metabolizes for excretion, allowing excessive amounts of medication to remain in the body over longer than normal periods of time. The rate of metabolism is especially important for the elderly, people with liver disease, and those with debilitating illnesses. The professional who is administering IV fluids/medications must be aware of these conditions and others that may affect metabolism, distribution, and excretion and monitor the patient accordingly.

Excretion of drugs occurs through respiration, perspiration, urination, and defecation. The rate of excretion is dependent on the chemical composition of the drug, the rate of metabolism, and route of administration. IV infusions will be absorbed, distributed, metabolized, and excreted faster than medications given orally or by other parenteral routes. Thus, some medications given intravenously must be administered more frequently.

IV PHARMACOLOGY RELATED TO BODY SYSTEMS

When looking in drug references most medications are found in alphabetical order by generic name. This is helpful when looking for a specific drug, but to aid in learning the implications of using drugs for IV therapy this text will provide general information related to drug classifications that are used by body systems or by those that affect the entire body. When using a specific medication that is either unknown or the information has not been used for a long period of time, the professional should use either a drug reference or drug insert to do the needed research to provide patient safety. Remember that drug dosages vary greatly even within the same classifications of medications, so this information must be drug specific at the time of administration.

IV Anti-Infective Agents

Anti-infective agents are perhaps the most frequently used of the IV medications, especially antibiotics. Anti-infectives include antibiotics, antifungals, and antiviral medications. Antibiotics may be either bacteriostatic, which inhibit bacterial growth by producing a defective cell wall, or bacteriocidal, which alters the growth of the microorganism itself. The primary contraindication to antibiotics is the prior history of hypersensitivity to the drug. The allergic reactions can be life threatening and, when given intravenously, may occur almost instantaneously. Another disadvantage includes the possibility of **superinfections** after prolonged used of the drug. Finally because some antibiotics have been used over long periods, some of the bacteria are now found to be drug resistant. Remember that the drug is not ineffective because of its action, but rather the bacteria does not respond to the specific medication and the microbe becomes more dangerous because of the ineffectiveness of the medications. One of the major problems is the inappropriate use of antibiotics for viral infections for which this classification is ineffective.

The professional administering IV anti-infective medications should know normal dosage for the drug, the side effects, and incompatibilities. Important also is to know the time the medication is stable after reconstitution if that is a factor in the administration. Being familiar with side effects and adverse reactions is important, and with antibiotics the professional should always be alert for drug sensitivity and possible anaphylaxis.

Antibiotics

Antibiotics are natural or synthetic substances that kill or inhibit the growth of microorganisms. Antibiotics are usually divided into different families of medications, such as penicillins, cephalosporins, tetracyclines, and others, by their action—**bacteriostatic** or **bactericidal**—and their actions against specific bacteria.

Penicillins

Penicillins are both natural and semisynthetic antibiotics that are derived from the fungus *Penicillium.* With the low cost, low toxicity, and good clinical efficacy, these antibiotics that are classified as bactericidal are often ordered when the microorganism is susceptible and the person is not allergic to the medication. The disadvantages to these medications are the possibility of phlebitis and its drug interactions with other antibiotics. Aminoglycosides cannot be delivered in the same container or tubing as penicillins. Procaine penicillins should never be given intravenously.

Penicillin G potassium (Pfizerpen), a natural penicillin, may be given either as continuous or intermittent IV therapy for bacteriocidal action. Because of being relatively nontoxic, although this medication does have hypersensitivity issues as with other penicillins, treatment of severe infections is one of the main indications for use. Hypersensitivity manifestations are similar to those found with all penicillins, such as dermatologically with rashes and urticaria; serum sickness–like reactions such as myalgia, fever, or malaise; hematologic reactions such as hemolytic anemia or leukopenia; and possibly anaphylaxis.

Second types of penicillin used intravenously are penicillinase-resistant penicillins such as methicillin sodium (Staphcillin). These penicillins are used to treat *Staphylococcus aureus* or *Staphylococcus epidermidis* infections. The side effects are similar to those found with natural penicillins. However, nafcillin sodium (Nafcil)

found in this category is more likely to cause phlebitis, although it does not cause as many kidney reactions.

Aminopenicillins, such as ampicillin sodium (Unipen or Totacillin-N), may be injected directly or by the more common means of an intermittent infusion. The stability of ampicillin after reconstitution is about 4 hours when added to a solution containing dextrose. However, if the medication is added to isotonic saline without dextrose, the time is extended to 8 hours. Finally, when placed in a minibag, the stability may last for 48 hours. A rash is the most common side effect of using this medication.

Some penicillins have extended or wider spectrums against microorganisms that have been identified by laboratory testing. Mezlocillin (Mezcil) and piperacillin (Pipracil) are typical of this group of antibiotics. These drugs have similar dermatologic and hematologic reactions to the other penicillins. Administration may be direct injection, **intermittent infusion,** or **continuous infusion.** It is important to follow the recommended rate of infusion and not exceed the flow rate because rapid infusion of some of this category of medications may result in seizures.

Cephalosporins

Cephalosporins are similar to the penicillins, having similar indications as bactericides, side effects, and contraindications. Cephalosporins are classified by spectrum rather than class. This group of medications has nephrotoxic effects and should not be given to a patient with hypersensitivity to penicillin. Cephalosporins are known to present a high risk for phlebitis so the infusion site should be observed and rotated frequently.

First-generation cephalosporins, such as cefazolin (Ancef and Kefzol) and cephradine (Anspor and Velosef), are used with such bacteria as *Staphylococcus* microorganisms. Used for severe infections of the many body systems, these drugs have similar side effects as penicillins, including anaphylaxis.

Second-generation cephalosporins include cefoxitin sodium (Mefoxin), cefamandole nafate

(Mandol), and cefotetan disodium (Cefotan). The side effects, actions, interactions, and contraindications are similar to those found with first-generation medications. The advantage for these medications is their usefulness with anaerobic microorganisms.

With the ability to cross the blood–brain barrier, third-generation cephalosporins are often used with neurologic infections. Again, these drugs have basically the same side effects, interactions, and contraindications as found in all generations of cephalosporins. Medications typical of this category are cefotaxime sodium (Claforan), ceftazidime (Fortaz and Tazidime), and ceftriaxone sodium (Rocephin). These are usually used in home care because the medication is given as one dose daily.

Fourth-generation cephalosporins, such as cefepime (Maxipime), are relatively new but are being accepted by the Food and Drug Administration (FDA) for use with severe infections, especially of the urinary tract, and for dermatologic conditions. The interactions, side effects, and allergic reactions are similar to other cephalosporins.

Aminoglycosides

Aminoglycosides, bactericidal agents, cause balance and hearing loss by damaging the 8th cranial nerve. Therefore, the patient receiving these medications over a period of time should be assessed for this adverse reaction. Another side effect is muscle weakness. The margin between therapeutic and toxic is small, but an advantage is the length of time the medication remains in the body for further therapeutic effect. Aminoglycosides such as gentamicin (Garamycin), amikacin sulfate (Amikin), and tobramycin sulfate (Nebcin and Tobrex) may be given as a single larger dose instead of the multiple daily doses. The single large dose administered over a period longer than 60 minutes seems to reduce the toxicity.

Tetracyclines

Tetracyclines, such as minocycline (Minocin), were the first broad-spectrum antibiotics and are considered both bactericidal and bacteriostatic,

depending on the dose administered. These drugs may be used when penicillin therapy is contraindicated. Photosensitive reactions may occur with tetracycline therapy so patients, especially those receiving therapy at home, should be informed to stay out of the sun and use sunscreen when outdoors. The infusion site should be rotated more frequently than every 48 hours because this classification of medications tends to cause venous irritation and thrombophlebitis. An intermittent infusion over a period of 1 to 4 hours is the most commonly used means of administration for tetracyclines.

Macrolides

Closely related to tetracyclines, **macrolides** are considered to be bacteriostatic and may have some bactericidal activity when administered in high dosages. Macrolides include erythromycin (only erythromycin lactobionate [Erythrocin] or erythromycin gluceptate [Ilotycin] can be administered intravenously) and azithromycin (Zithromax). These medications tend to cause phlebitis and must be diluted in at least 100 mL of solvent such as normal saline or 5% dextrose solutions and given over a relatively long period of time. Dilution and rotating the site make these medications less irritating for the patient. These medications are considered to be relatively free of serious side effects, so they are considered one of the safest for patients. Macrolides are used for staphylococcal, streptococcal, and pneumococcal infections as an alternative for patients who are allergic to penicillin.

Chloramphenicol

Chloramphenicol (Chloromycetin) is found in ophthalmic and IV forms for use with serious infections. This medication is administered by intermittent infusion and may be administered concurrently with penicillin G for serious anaerobic infections. Because of the potential for serious and potentially fatal reactions, chloramphenicol should not be used unless no other medication is effective. Because of the toxicity of this medication, the patient must be closely monitored when this medication is administered.

Fluroquinolones

A relatively new class of antibiotics is the **fluoroquinolones**, which include such drugs as ciprofloxacin (Cipro), levofloxacin (Levaquin), gatifloxacin (Tequin), and ofloxacin (Floxin). These medications are bactericidal in gram-positive and gram-negative organisms, and with large doses they are effective with anaerobic microorganisms. Additional patient hydration is needed because these medications tend to crystallize in urine. For the patient at home, photosensitivity could be a side effect. Because most of the medications require only once-a-day dosing, these drugs are often given intermittently with home infusion for convenience, and in hospital settings to reduce the damage to veins.

Other Antibiotics

Other antibiotics such as vancomycin (Vancocin), clindamycin (Cleocin), lincomycin (Lincocin), and others that are introduced on a regular basis to reduce the chance of bacteria resistance. Before administering any of these medications, as should be done with all medications, be sure to read the literature for the proper time of administration as well as the side effects and adverse reactions. Remember that patient safety is of utmost consideration and importance.

Antifungals

Two antifungals most frequently administered intravenously are amphotericin B (Fungazone) and fluconazole (Diflucan), with amphotericin being the medication used most frequently. Antifungals, used to treat fungal infections, are suspensions, and most should be administered using an in-line filter as directed by the manufacturer. Some of these medications should be administered without a filter because of the suspension state of the drug. Following manufacturer's instructions is of utmost importance for patient safety and drug effectiveness. The infusion should run for 2 to 6 hours, using the most distal vein available to prevent irritation of the veins proximal to the body. Rapid infusion may cause circulatory collapse, a danger with these medications. These drugs should not be added to saline solution because a precipitate will form. These medications should be used only in a hospital situation because of frequently occurring side effects, such as nausea and vomiting, headache, chills, fever, malaise, and anorexia. Thrombophlebitis is an expected adverse reaction when these medications are administered, but the physician may decrease this possibility by ordering heparin to be added to the fluids. Amphotericin B is light sensitive and should not be mixed with any other drugs because of the numerous incompatibilities. Fluconazole must be administered in a glass container and should not have other medications added to the container. Careful, more frequent monitoring of the patient is essential with these medications.

Antivirals

Used to treat viral diseases, antivirals, such as acyclovir (Zovirax), ganciclovir, (Cytovene) and cidofovir (Vistide), must be used after a patient has been prehydrated to prevent renal toxicity. These medications prevent the replication of viruses. A safe broad-spectrum antiviral drug has not been discovered. These antivirals are given as intermittent infusions two to three times a day. Headaches and thrombophlebitis are common adverse reactions even if the medication is infused over a period of at least 1 hour. Patient output should be carefully monitored when administering antivirals intravenously. These medications are incompatible with blood products and other medications because of the alkaline pH.

Antiretrovirals

Antiretrovirals are administered intravenously only until oral therapy can be initiated and the necessary blood levels achieved. These medications must run over a period of at least 1 hour at a constant rate and should be diluted in D-5-W or normal saline. These medications, which include zidovudine (Retrovir), have many drug incompatibilities that should be checked prior to adding to fluids containing other medications.

Sulfonamides

Sulfonamides, such as trimethoprim-sulfamethoxazole (Bactrim, Septra), have been used for more than 50 years to treat infections, especially those of the urinary tract. These medications inhibit growth and reproduction of the microorganism and are administered as intermittent infusions of up to 3 to 4 doses daily. Found in combination of sulfonamide and another drug, the precautions found with the sulfonamides must be followed. The common signs of hypersensitivity are found with these medications.

IV Medications for the Central Nervous System

Drugs for the central nervous system (CNS) most frequently administered intravenously are analgesics. Other types of medications may include sedatives; hypnotics; and some that are specific to the nervous system, such as anticonvulsants.

Analgesics

Analgesics are used for pain management. Prior to infusing any analgesic the patient should be assessed for the location of the pain; its intensity, quality, frequency, onset, and duration; and any aggravating or alleviating factors. Parenteral dosing may be by continuous infusion or by intermittent routes. Continuous infusion provides continuous levels of pain control without the peaks of side effects or breakthrough pain. Intermittent dosing can be accomplished by **patient-controlled analgesia (PCA)** or through direct injection of the medication into the IV line at the time analgesia is needed.

Controlled Substance Analgesics

Controlled analgesics, previously called **narcotics,** are used to control different levels of pain. Prior to administration of analgesics, the pain should be evaluated so the properly indicated controlled analgesic may be administered because

in many instances the physician will order more than one analgesic or different doses of medications for different levels of pain.

The most commonly used controlled analgesic medication for continuous IV use is morphine. Other controlled analgesics include meperidine (Demerol) and hydromorphone (Dilaudid). The main indications for these types of medications, and especially morphine, are the pain of coronary occlusion, chronic pain of malignancies, and acute pain following surgery. Most analgesics are potentiated by other central nervous system depressants, neuromuscular blockers, adrenergic blockers, phenothiazines, and MAOIs (monoamine oxidase inhibitors). Care with obtaining a full patient history is important to prevent adverse reactions from drug interactions. Morphine should never be given full strength; it should be diluted prior to administration.

Morphine may be administered by slow direct injection or by continuous infusion. The major side effect is respiratory depression; patients with respiratory disease must be carefully monitored. Other side effects include nausea, tachycardia, hypotension, vomiting, constipation, cardiac depression, and coma.

Hydromorphone (Dilaudid) is 5 to 10 times more potent than morphine, whereas meperidine (Demerol) has about 20% of the analgesic potency and a shorter duration of action. These two medications also require the same safety measures as found with morphine. These two medications should also be diluted prior to infusing, and patients should be evaluated prior to administration, during the administration, and following the infusion in the same manner as with morphine. Because of interactions, the use of hydromorphone in IV tubing should be assessed prior to administration.

The **antagonist** for narcotic analgesics is naloxone (Narcan). The mode of action is to block the opiate receptors and thus inhibit or reverse the narcotic effect.

Opiate Agonists–Antagonists

Opiate agonists–antagonists include pentazocine (Talwin), nalbuphine (Nubain), and butorphanol

(Stadol). These medications may be administered undiluted, as an **IV injections (IV push),** and have lower addictive levels than found with the opiate and **opioid** medications (narcotics). When these medications are given to a patient who has not previously received a narcotic analgesic, the medication behaves as an agonist, acting much like a narcotic analgesic. However, when administered when the patient is receiving a narcotic analgesic, these medications have an antagonist effect and inhibit the response of the narcotic. These medications are used with moderate to severe pain but have the advantage of being low in addictive tendencies. As with narcotics, these medications potentiate CNS depressants such as tranquilizers and sedatives. Side effects include dizziness, vertigo, headache, euphoria, confusion, and insomnia.

Sedatives, Hypnotics, and Anxiolytics

CNS depressants are used to cause drowsiness (sedatives), induce sleep (hypnotics), and relieve anxiety (anxiolytics). These may provide levels of sedation from mild sedation to anesthesia.

Barbituates

Barbiturates are drugs that produce any sedation from mild to hypnosis and even coma. Included in this category are phenobarbital (Luminal), amobarbital (Amytal), secobarbital (Seconal), and thiopental (Pentothal), with the main difference between each of these drugs being the time of onset and duration. Depending on the indication for the use of the medication, barbiturates may be administered either as intermittent or one-time dose for sedation or as continuous administration for such conditions as status epilepticus. These medications have interactions with other medications, so prior to administration intravenously, the interactions should be known. The most commonly seen side effects include respiratory depression, hypotension, and excessive sedation. Adverse reactions include pain at the infusion site and, more importantly, the tendency to thrombophlebitis.

Benzodiazepines

Benzodiazepines are different medications from barbiturates but are often used for the same indications. These medications reduce anxiety, produce sedation, relax muscle spasticity, and act as anticonvulsants. The common drugs in this classification are diazepam (Valium), lorazepam (Ativan), and midazolam hydrochloride (Versed). Midazolam, a short-acting drug, has been used for conscious sedation for such minor surgical procedures as endoscopy or as a preoperative sedative. Lorazepam should be diluted with either D-5-W or normal saline for immediate administration directly into the vein or should be given as close to the terminal end of the tubing as possible. Adding these drugs to other fluids is not indicated. These medications may potentiate other depressants. Side effects include drowsiness, ataxia, confusion, syncope, and vertigo. Apnea, hypotension, and bradycardia also are possible.

The preferred method of administration of diazepam is directly into the vein because of the possible precipitation of the medication within the plastic tubing. If given into tubing, the medication should be given as close to the vein as possible and flushed with normal saline prior to and after the administration.

Promethazine (Phenergan) may be given to potentiate sedative properties and to assist with the prevention of nausea and vomiting. With patients with terminal illnesses, it may also be given to assist with pain control. This medication is irritating to the veins and will cause phlebitis. Therefore, the peripheral venous access should be rotated often when promethazine is administered on a regular basis.

Anticonvulsants

Other reasons for use of CNS medications include convulsions that are treated with anticonvulsants. Many of the drugs already discussed are used for this purpose, although there are specific drugs for this condition. Phenytoin (Dilantin) is one of the specific anticonvulsants used. This medication precipitates if the pH is changed; therefore the tubing must be flushed with normal saline prior to and after administration. Normal saline in the amounts of 25 to 50 mL may be used for dilution with each 100 mg of phenytoin; however, the greatest dilution should be 100 mg per 100 mL of solvent. The IV solution should be prepared just prior to administration, and the infusion should be added above the filter with the infusion time to be within an hour.

Magnesium sulfate is another medication used as an anticonvulsant that is given intravenously with preeclampsia and eclampsia to prevent seizures. This medication may be administered by IV injection or by intermittent infusion over 4 hours. The onset of action when administered intravenously is almost immediate and lasts for about 30 minutes.

IV Medications for the Cardiovascular System

Drugs given for use with the cardiovascular system include those that affect cardiac strength and cardiac rhythm and those that are used to reverse hypotension, to control hypertension, and to improve blood flow. The following is only a summary of the medications because the use in this area is specialized and beyond the scope of this text.

Alpha–Beta-Adrenergic Agonists

Alpha–beta-adrenergic agonists, such as epinephrine (Adrenalin), imitate the responses of the sympathetic nervous system by elevating systolic blood pressure, lowering diastolic blood pressure, and increasing the strength of the cardiac contraction and the contraction rate, thus increasing cardiac output. This medication may be given as a bolus in emergency situations, as an intravenous injection, or as an infusion. When given as an overdose or too rapidly the patient may have symptoms that occur with the stimulation of the sympathetic nervous system. If the medication **extravasates,** severe tissue damage may occur because of its vasoconstriction properties. Epinephrine interacts with many drugs, including the potentiation of anesthetics and antihistamines.

Alpha-Adrenergic Agents

The alpha-adrenergic classification of medications is used for vasoconstriction and for cardiac stimulation, usually with hypotension. The most commonly used medication is metaraminol bitartrate (Aramine), a drug that strengthens cardiac contractility and increases blood flow to essential body organs, such as brain, kidneys, and heart, and mimics naturally occurring norepinephrine. After the emergency situation has passed and the hypotensive state is stabilized, metaraminol bitartrate may be given by continuous infusion. During continuous infusion the patient's blood pressure should be monitored closely. If the infusion extravasates, the tissue will be damaged, necrose, and slough.

Beta-Adrenergic Agonists

Beta-adrenergic agonists, such as dopamine (Inotropin) or isoproterenol (Isuprel), act to stimulate the heart and dilate the bronchi. These medications stimulate the contractility of the heart and increase cardiac output, blood pressure, and urinary output. Therefore this medication is used to treat shock. Dopamine may be administered as a continuous infusion with blood pressure monitored frequently. Side effects related to bradycardia, tachycardia, hypertension, hypotension, and vasoconstriction include nausea, vomiting, headache, and dyspnea.

Beta-Adrenergic Blockers

Propranolol hydrochloride (Inderal) is a typical beta-adrenergic blocker that impedes the action of norepinephrine and epinephrine. These medications have an antiarrhythmic effect and are used to treat arrhythmias such as paroxysmal atrial tachycardia, atrial flutter, and atrial fibrillation. Given as a slow IV injection, side effects include syncope, vertigo, and visual disturbances.

Cardiac Glycosides

Cardiac glycosides, such as digoxin (Lanoxin), are used to increase cardiac contractility and to alter the generation and conduction of electrical impulse to increase cardiac output and to slow the rate of contractions. Used to treat atrial fibrillation, congestive heart failure, and paroxysmal tachycardia, digoxin has a narrow margin for safety between the therapeutic dose and the toxic amount. The drug is given either diluted with sterile water, D-5-W, or normal saline for infusion or undiluted by IV injection, and it may be repeated intermittently until the digitalizing dose is obtained. Early common signs of toxicity are nausea, vomiting, and anorexia with headaches, blurred vision, changed color vision, confusion, and diarrhea being later signs of toxicity. Because so many drugs interact with digoxin, all medications that the patient is taking should be evaluated prior to the initiation of the IV therapy.

Antidysrhythmics

Cardiac antidysrhythmics are used when a deviation in the normal sinus rhythm occurs to prevent or stop an irregular heartbeat or rhythm. No single drug is typical for this group, but several are used for various causes of arrhythmias. Some antiarrhythmics, such as quinidine gluconate and procainamide hydrochloride (Pronestyl), are used to decrease the amount of sodium that is transported through the heart tissue, thus slowing the conduction of the electrical impulse through the AV (atrioventricular) node. The side effects are acute hypotension, diaphoresis, tinnitus, and visual disturbances. Care must be taken with patients who are also taking digoxin.

Another group of antidysrhythmics promotes uniform conduction rates by decreasing the refractory period of the Purkinje fibers and the ventricular myocardium. This group includes lidocaine that is given either as a bolus in the amount of 50 to 100 mg at a rate not exceeding 25 mg/min. The bolus dose may be repeated but then the medication would be given as a continuous infusion at the rate of 1 to 4 mg/min. The second commonly used medication is phenytoin sodium (Dilantin), which is used when the arrhythmia is digitalis induced. These drugs have little margin for error. Patient sedation and

drowsiness are expected, but high blood levels may lead to unconsciousness and respiratory distress. The more commons side effects are lightheadedness, apprehension, blurred vision, and numbness.

Another group, such as propranolol hydrochloride (Inderal) that is a typical beta blocker, may be used for arrhythmias. See the earlier information about these medications.

The antidysrhythmics used to slow the electrical impulse by blocking the calcium influx into the cardiac cells include verapamil hydrochloride (Isoptin) and diltiazem (Cardizem). Severe hypotension may occur with these drugs; side effects include dizziness, headache, abdominal pain, and either bradycardia or tachycardia. If given with digoxin, the patient must be monitored closely because these medications have potentiating interactions. Both medications have other interactions that must be closely monitored.

Other medications are available for use as antidysrhythmics but are not as commonly used as those discussed earlier.

IV Hematology Agents

Anticoagulants and thrombolytics are used to keep the body in homeostasis by maintaining the coagulation factors in the blood within normal limits. If the blood tends to clot or has a treatment that could initiate a clot, an anticoagulant may be used. However, if the patient is bleeding and the clotting time needs to be shortened, a thrombolytic may be prescribed.

Anticoagulants

Anticoagulants interfere with the coagulation or clotting of blood to prevent thrombosis. In the medical setting, these may also be used to reduce the risk of a clot formation. A commonly used anticoagulant is heparin sodium, which in small doses inhibits the conversion of prothrombin to thrombin. Heparin is often used in the prevention of venous thrombi and pulmonary emboli, found with renal dialysis; in the prevention of clotting during cardiac and arterial surgery, and in the treatment of myocardial infarctions. To provide a constant degree of anticoagulation, heparin is often given as a continuous infusion, although it may be given as an intermittent injection. A coagulation time is necessary prior to the therapy and throughout therapy at regular intervals. The most common side effect is bleeding and hemorrhage as a result of increased bleeding times, although bleeding from the gums, gastrointestinal tract, and nose are often signs of elevated prothrombin times. Heparin interacts with many medications, so a careful check of the drug regimen for the patient is necessary to prevent adverse reactions. Finally, heparin also is used as an IV flush to retain patency of IV lines and prevent the development of small thrombi during intermittent infusions.

Thrombolytic Agents

The opposite of anticoagulants are thrombolytic agents, such as streptokinase (Streptase), used to dissolve an already formed clot or thrombi. By degrading fibrinogen and fibrin clots, streptokinase causes lysis of coronary artery thrombi, pulmonary emboli, and deep-vessel thrombi. The side effects are bleeding, fever, and hypersensitivity. For the older person with diabetes mellitus, this therapy tends to cause more complications.

IV Drugs for Fluid and Electrolyte Balance

Fluid and electrolyte balance was discussed in Chapter 2. To maintain homeostasis that has been compromised due to medical conditions, medications may be required to correct acid–base balances, to excrete extra fluids from the body, or to replace or maintain electrolyte or fluid levels. In many cases, these are the drugs that are used for maintenance therapy and the patient remains on continuous infusions throughout a hospital stay. The replacement of electrolytes and fluids may also be a reason for IV therapy on an ambulatory-care basis when an acute condition is the indication for immediate IV therapy.

Medications Used to Correct Acid–Base Imbalances

When metabolic alkalosis occurs, acidifying agents will be used to reverse the alkaline state. Acidifying agents will react with the alkaline ions to form water that is excreted by the body to bring the person back into homeostasis from the state of imbalance. In this case, the patient must be watched for respiratory distress, irregular heartbeats, headache, and disorientation.

If the body becomes acidic, alkalinizing agents, such as sodium bicarbonate, will be administered to reduce the electrolyte imbalance. Sodium bicarbonate reacts with many medications so the drugs being taken must be carefully assessed prior to starting this medication. Because of the many incompatibilities with other drugs, the IV tubing must be flushed both prior to and after any infusion of the acidic medications. If the medication extravasates into the tissue, severe tissue damage with necrosis and ulceration may occur. The rate of flow must not be rapid because complications such as cerebral hemorrhage may occur.

Diuretics

Loop and thiazide diuretics may be administered intravenously. Diuretics increase the amount of water eliminated through the kidneys and are used to treat severe edema including that from cardiac and nephrotic conditions.

Loop diuretics, such as furosemide (Lasix), inhibit the reabsorption of fluids in the loop of Henle to remove excess fluid from the body. Large doses of furosemide should be infused at a slow rate, whereas doses of 20 to 40 mg may be infused as a direct injection over 1 to 2 minutes. Hypotension and tinnitus are side effects, and this medication interacts with other medications, especially those that cause nephrotoxicity.

Thiazide diuretics, such as chlorothiazide sodium (Diuril), interfere with the reabsorption of sodium in the distal convoluted tubules. This medication is not as effective as the loop diuretics but is used with toxemias and diabetes insipidus. Because of the potency of chlorothiazide, the oral route of administration is preferable.

IV Drugs for Electrolyte Replacements

Electrolytes are replaced by using IV fluids when the specific deficiency is known. The most common electrolytes that need replacement are calcium and potassium.

Calcium is most commonly replaced using calcium gluconate that is administered as a continuous infusion. The side effects include flushing, bradycardia, tingling, and depressed neuromuscular function. This may also be given as a direct injection at a rate of 0.5 mL over a minute.

When replacing potassium, either potassium chloride or potassium phosphate most often are used. Loss of potassium most frequently occurs following diuretic therapy, vomiting, diarrhea, and acidosis. This medication does cause vein irritation so the amount of medication per liter should not exceed 80 mEq. Under no circumstance should potassium be infused undiluted because this may lead to cardiac arrest.

IV Hormones

Several hormones are given intravenously such as corticosteroids for use with immunosuppressive or malignant diseases. The adverse effects are not readily seen but are a result of long-term therapy.

Estrogens

Estrogens are given intravenously to treat breast cancer and for prostatic enlargement. These medications, such as diethylstilbestrol (Stilphostrol), are given intermittently over a period of days with the rate of each infusion increased after the first 15 minutes. This medication should always be diluted in at least 300 mL of fluids prior to administration.

Insulin

Insulin, used to treat diabetes mellitus, acts as a catalyst for carbohydrate metabolism by allowing the transport of glucose and allowing its use in peripheral tissues. Regular insulin may be given intravenously and may be used for emergency treatment of hyperglycemic reactions.

The potency of the insulin that is given to the patient may be affected by the absorption of the medication in the tubing and IV solution containers. Insulin may be administered as a direct injection or a continuous infusion. The amount of insulin depends on the medical condition of the patient and the reason for the administration. This medication does potentiate anticoagulants, salicylates, sulfonamides, and tetracycline.

TOTAL PARENTERAL NUTRITION

Total parenteral nutrition (TPN) is usually administered through peripherally inserted central catheter (PICC) lines but may be infused into peripheral veins, although these fluids tend to be irritating to peripheral veins. The nutritional components of fats, proteins, carbohydrates, electrolytes, vitamins, and minerals are determined by the medical condition of the patient, the type of malnutrition, and the cause of nutritional deficiency.

In this section the standard solutions for TPN and the care of the peripheral veins with these fluids will be discussed. The actual fluid components are multiple, with many combinations to meet the patient's needs, and are beyond the scope of this text.

Peripheral parenteral nutrition (PPN) is used to supplement feedings and has fewer complications than when given through a central line. However, these fluids contain fewer calories and less protein because a lower concentration must be used. The typical fluid contains an isotonic, high-calorie fat emulsion, including dextrose, amino acids, electrolytes, vitamins, and trace elements, that may be infused into the peripheral veins. The dextrose and lipids provide energy, whereas the amino acids meet the patient's needs for protein. The fats and lipids also provide the caloric needs for enzyme reactions at the cellular level. The dextrose level for dilution of these fluids may be 2.5%, 5%, or 10%, but the osmolarity of the solutions should be less than 600 mOsm/L. Medications that are compatible, such as heparin to prevent thrombophlebitis, may be added to these fluids.

The use of TPN in peripheral veins is usually short term, for 5 to 14 days, but if a longer term is necessary, a central line should be considered. Even with the reduced concentration of the nutritional elements, phlebitis and infiltration into the surrounding tissue are frequent problems. Because of the damage to tissues and veins, the placement of the catheter should be evaluated prior to infusion and confirmed to prevent unnecessary trauma.

Remember that these fluids have short expiration times and should be used immediately. If storage is necessary, refrigeration should be used, but the fluids should be removed 60 minutes before the time for administration to allow fluids to warm to room temperature. After 24 hours, these fluids should be discarded to prevent the possibility of bacterial contamination.

INCOMPATIBILITIES OF FLUIDS AND MEDICATIONS

In some instances the IV fluids have incompatibilities with medications. Factors that affect drug administration include solubility and compatibility, such as drug administration type of administration set, pH of the fluids and medications, and duration of drug/drug or drug/solution contact. Fluids containing dextrose are slightly acidic and should be used with slightly acidic medications, whereas saline solutions are slightly alkaline and should be used with slightly alkaline medications. Several of the antibiotics on the market require an acidic fluid for dilution because the medication is not stable when not placed in an acidic environment.

Drugs may be compatible in some solutions and incompatible with other solutions. The incompatibility may be prevalent when two or more medications are mixed or when specific medications are mixed in incompatible fluids. Finally, incompatibilities may occur as a result of the tubing and drugs that are absorbed or changed by specific tubing materials. These incompatibilities should be detected by pharmacists in inpatient settings but may become the responsibility of the person

initiating the IV therapy in other medical or outpatient environments. When in doubt of incompatibilities, check the medication reference materials and, for safety, flush the IV administration set with saline prior to and after medications are infused.

Some medications interact with the plastic flexible IV bags because of the polyvinyl chloride (PVC) found therein. These drugs include vitamin A acetate, insulin, warfarin, and phenothiazine tranquilizers.

Incompatibility may also occur when mixing medications because of physical properties of the drugs. Insolubility, created when a drug is added to an inappropriate fluid, is the incomplete solution or the forming of a precipitate. This is more common with multiple additives but may occur when the products being mixed interact. Usually a visible precipitate occurs. The presence of calcium in a medication often indicates that a precipitate will develop when mixing two or more medications in IV fluids. Because Ringer's solutions contain calcium, always check for incompatibilities when using this solution.

Table 7–1 is provided as a guide when fluid/drug incompatibilities need to be evaluated. It is not intended to cover all possible incompatibilities, but it does provide basic knowledge for the more frequently prescribed fluids or medications.

SAFETY CONSIDERATIONS

Patient safety with the administration of medications is always the foremost consideration. Therefore, because IV medications cannot be reversed once administered, special care must be taken with IV administration of medications to ensure this safety. Some of the steps that will assist with this include the following:

• Always be cognizant of the medication that is ordered, normal dosage, side effects, and compatibilities. Be aware of the reconstitution strength and the necessary dilution of the medication, and ensure that proper storage has occurred prior to administering the medications. Remember the person administering the medication is responsible for patient safety.

Table 7-1 COMMON FLUID/DRUG INCOMPATIBILITIES*

Drug	D5W	D5	D5 S	NS	R	LR	Other
Amphotericin B		x	x	x		x	
Ampicillin	x		x		x	x	
Amsacrine			x				
Cefamandole					x	x	Check all cephalosporins
Cefotetan			x		x	x	
Cefoxitin			x				
Cephapirin					x	x	
Cephradine					x	x	
Chlordiazepoxide HCl				x	x	x	
Ciprofloxin					x	x	
Diazepam	x		x	x	x		
Dopamine					x		
Doxycycline			x		x	x	
Erythromycin	x		x		x	x	Check chemical base
Fat emulsion	x			x			
Gentamicin					x	x	
Kanamycin			x		x	x	
K-phosphate					x	x	
Levarterenol		x		x			
Mannitol		x	x	x			
Methicillin					x	x	
Methylprednisone sodium succinate				x			
Nitroglycerin					x	x	
Norepinephrine				x	x		
Oxytetracycline						x	
Phenytoin	x		x	x	x	x	
Piperacillin					x		
Procainamide	x						
Sodium bicarbonate	x					x	
Thiopental						x	
Vitamin B$_{12}$	x						
Warfarin sodium	x		x			x	

*"x" in box indicates an incompatibility
D-5-W, Dextrose 5% in water
D-5-1/2 NS, Dextrose 5% in 0.45% normal saline
D-5-S, Dextrose 5% in normal saline
NS, 0.9% sodium chloride or normal saline
R, Ringer's solution
LR, lactated Ringer's solution

- Do a safety check for expiration dates, leaks, or loss of patency of the fluid container or tubing.
- Evaluate the patient's medical record for possibilities of hypersensitivity to the fluids or the added medications.
- Use strict aseptic technique in all steps of the administration.
- After initiating fluid administration, evaluate the patient often for side effects and adverse reactions. Take proper safety measures as indicated.

- Check the infusion rates regularly to ensure that therapeutic levels of the medication are being provided and the rate of infusion is that ordered by the physician.
- Always be aware that anaphylaxis is a possibility even with the least toxic fluids or medications.

Medications are given for other indications such as chemotherapy and PCA. These indications are not in the scope of this text because of the more advanced educational levels and the resultant techniques necessary for patient safety.

REVIEW QUESTIONS

1. What are the four processes of pharmacokinetics?
2. What process of pharmacokinetics is not used in IV therapy and why?
3. Name four areas of patient assessment that are important to provide patient safety with the administration of IV medications.
4. What is the difference in a side effect and an adverse reaction?
5. The absorption rate with IV therapy is slow and therefore not dangerous to the patient. Is this statement true or false? Explain your answer.
6. What classification of medications is most frequently administered by IV infusion?
7. What are the three main classifications of anti-infective medications that are given intravenously?
8. What are the three main dangers of giving anti-infective medications over prolonged periods of time?
9. Which penicillins should not be administered intravenously?
10. Why should antifungals be administered with an in-line filter?
11. Why is it important to initiate IV therapy in distal veins when the drug has a side effect of phlebitis?
12. What is a bolus of medication? What is an IV injection of medication?
13. What are the IV uses of heparin?
14. What type of nutritional components are found in TPN?
15. Why must PPN be used only for short-term treatment of nutritional needs of the patient?

Chapter 8

Starting an Intravenous Infusion

Chapter Outline

Order for IV Therapy and Assess Patient

Gathering of Equipment

Preparation of the Patient

Preparation of the Equipment

Selecting a Suitable Site

Steps in the Initiation of IV Infusion Therapy

Care, Assessment, and Maintenance of the Infusion Site

Replacement of the Ordered Fluids and Medications

Discontinuation of IV Therapy

Learning Objectives

Upon successful completion of this chapter, the student will be able to:

- Identify the equipment and supplies needed to initiate IV therapy as ordered by the medical professional.
- Assemble the equipment necessary to prepare to perform the venipuncture.
- Select and prepare the proper site for IV therapy.
- Consider appropriate site selections related to rapid infusion, other needs for venous access, and patient comfort.

- Develop knowledge of the skills of venipuncture needed to initiate IV infusion therapy.
- Understand the care, assessment, and maintenance of the infusion site during infusion therapy and the replacement of the fluids and medications, as ordered.
- Perform the discontinuation of IV therapy, including dressings and assessment of site.

Key Terms

heparin lock—IV port that makes possible intermittent IV drug administration. The port or sterile hub is attached to the venipuncture device after its insertion into the vein and is filled with a heparin solution to maintain patency of the venous site.

macrodrip set—IV administration set with tubing that supplies large drops of fluids, such as 8 to 20 drops/mL.

microdrip set—IV administration set with tubing that supplies small drops of fluids, such as 50 to 60 drops/mL.

saline lock—IV port that makes possible intermittent IV drug administration. The port or sterile hub is attached to the venipuncture device after its insertion into the vein and is filled with normal saline to maintain patency of the site.

venipuncture device—needle used to puncture the skin and enter the vein when starting an IV; catheter may be left within vein for infusion therapy.

Intravenous (IV) therapy is used for many medical reasons, and patient safety is always of utmost importance when this therapy is performed. The actual procedure for initiating the infusion of fluids is basically that used for venipuncture, with additional threading of the infusion device into the vein. The use of IV therapy has increased in recent years and patient safety has been improved by the continuous improvement of IV supplies and pump technology. What was essentially an inpatient procedure in the recent past has become a therapeutic measure now found in ambulatory care. In either setting, the equipment, supplies, initiation, and care of the infusion site, as well as assessment of the patient throughout the procedure, are the same no matter where the infusion therapy occurs.

The initiation of IV therapy requires several considerations. The first step, as in all pharmacologic procedures, is to confirm the physician's order. A review of the patient's history is necessary, appropriate, and valuable. Hands are sanitized, as before any procedure. Supplies and equipment are assembled and transported to the patient's location, and the identity of the patient is confirmed verbally and by electronic detection systems as appropriate at the site of employment. In most situations, patient assessment is performed to establish a baseline for future assessments. The procedure should be explained to the patient and the patient made comfortable. The equipment is assembled, the potential venipuncture site is assessed, the skin is prepared, and then the venipuncture procedure is performed. Following the venipuncture, a dressing is applied to the site, the tubing is stabilized, and the patient is observed for tolerance of the procedure. During the infusion process, the patient and the infusion site need to be assessed frequently, and when the infusion is complete, the IV is discontinued. After the **venipuncture device** is removed, the site should be observed for possible complications. Once the procedure is complete and the patient appears stable, he or she receives care according to the physician's order. Documentation of the procedure must be completed (Figure 8–1).

ORDER FOR IV THERAPY AND ASSESS PATIENT

The first steps in initiating an IV are to check the physician's order and confirm the identity of the patient. The physician order is checked for the following:
- Patient's name
- IV solution
- Any medication to be added to the solution
- Amount of solution to be infused
- Time over which solution is to be infused or the time appropriate for the number of milliliters

Review the patient's history prior to initiating the infusion as circumstances allow (or if an emergency exists). This evaluation process provides the clinician with information regarding the patient's general health status as well as the rationale for the IV therapy. Helpful information to obtain includes the following:
- Information about the patient's present illness. This may help to assess how his or her fluid balance may be affected by the IV therapy and the expected results of therapy.
- Medication or other treatment the patient is receiving.
- The patient's ability to take oral fluids and nutrition.
- The relationship of fluid intake and output.
- Dietary restrictions.

The hand sanitization procedure is performed as the first step in infection control because this technique helps to remove microbes on the clinician's hands (Figure 8–2).

GATHERING OF EQUIPMENT

The next step in preparing for IV therapy is to assemble the proper equipment for initiating the IV infusion.

Correct Solution and Amount

The container of solution selected must be carefully checked against the prescriber's order for type of solution and the prescribed amount. The pharmacist in an inpatient setting will prepare

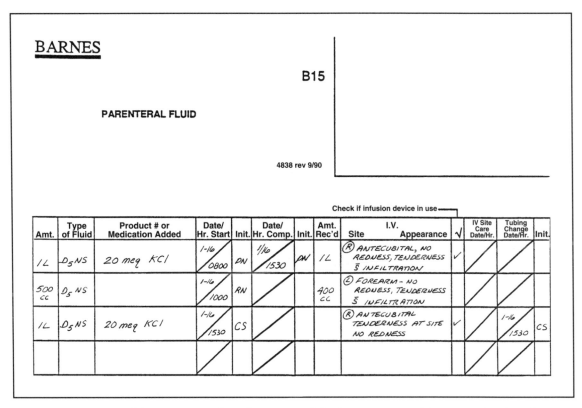

Figure 8-1   Example of documentation form for parenteral fluids. (From Perry AG, Potter PA: *Clinical nursing skills & techniques,* ed 6, St Louis, 2006, Mosby.)

the ordered fluids in most instances, whereas, in an ambulatory care, the person initiating the therapy may be responsible for selection of the IV fluids ordered. In some facilities, the pharmacy may send the administration set with the pharmacy order for fluids. Even if the set comes with the fluids, the person initiating the infusion should check the tubing, administration set, and fluids for accuracy to the physician's order, because the person administering the fluids is ultimately responsible for the infusion (Figure 8–3).

Correct Solution Administration Set or Tubing

Each type of solution may require special administration sets. It is best to check with a

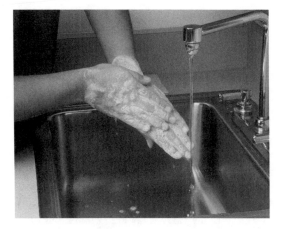

Figure 8-2   Handwashing. (From Young AP, Kennedy DB: Kinn's: *The medical assistant: an applied learning approach*, ed 9, St Louis, 2003, Saunders.)

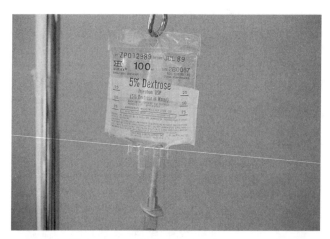

Figure 8-3 IV fluid container that should be used with an order for 100 mL D-5-W. (From Perry AG, Potter PA: *Clinical nursing skills & techniques,* ed 6, St Louis, 2006, Mosby.)

pharmacist, if available, about the type of administration set required when drugs have been added to the solution. If a pharmacist is not available, be sure the order contains the desired flow rate. Also, the prescribed rate will dictate if a **microdrip set** or a **macrodrip set** is indicated (Figure 8–4). Additionally, the use of an

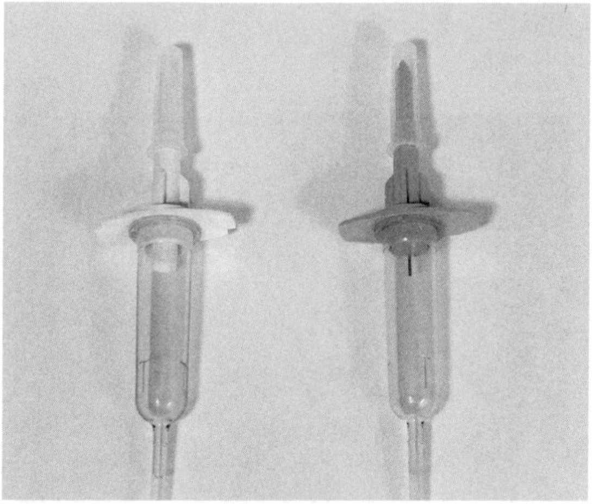

Figure 8-4   Left, IV macrodrip set. **Right,** Microdrip set. (From Leahy JM, Kizilay PE: *Foundations of nursing practice: a nursing process approach,* Philadelphia, 1998, Saunders.)

infusion device or pump will require special tubing that is used with that specific pump. Refer to Chapter 4 for additional information on equipment.

Antiseptic Solutions and Applicators

Antiseptic solutions and applicators are necessary for cleansing and disinfecting the skin at the proposed infusion site. The usual antiseptic solutions include 70% isopropyl alcohol, iodophor (iodine preparation), and chlorhexidine gluconate or others may be used depending on the protocol of the facility or the preference of the health provider.

Venipuncture/Infusion Devices

Infusion devices include over-the-needle catheters, butterfly needles, and through-the-needle catheters. An adequate supply of venipuncture devices in various types and sizes should be gathered and placed in a tray to carry them to the location of the patient. Antiseptic solutions and a selection of possible tourniquets should also be available. This adequate supply of infusion devices and compression articles prevents having to leave the patient's environment to obtain additional

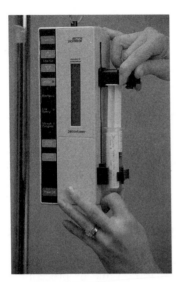

Figure 8-5   Mini-infusion pump. (From Perry AG, Potter PA: *Clinical nursing skills & techniques*, ed 6, St Louis, 2006, Mosby.)

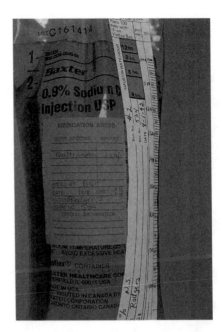

Figure 8-6   IV fluid bag with measurement tape. (From Perry AG, Potter PA: *Clinical nursing skills & techniques,* ed 6, St Louis, 2006, Mosby.)

supplies if needed. Remember, supplies should be a sufficient quantity to allow for contamination and a sufficient size to provide as painless a venipuncture as possible for the type of infusion ordered.

Devices for Regulation of Fluid Flow

Different types of infusion devices are available. The clinician should be familiar with what is available in the facility and understand how each works (Figure 8–5). The regulation device should be set for the flow rate, but the actual infusion rate should be evaluated on a regular basis. Refer to Chapter 4 for additional information concerning types of infusion regulation devices available for use.

Measurement Tapes for Marking Flow Rates

When an infusion device is not being used, the measurement tapes are applied to the bag or bottle of solution (Figure 8–6). These tapes indicate the time line for the fluid infusion and allow the health care professional responsible for the infusion therapy to check that the fluids are

flowing at the correct rate. Remember, this does not provide an entirely accurate flow rate, but rather an estimation. The volume of fluids infused should be checked and compared to the physician's order on a regular basis.

Appropriate Device for Holding Solution Container

Various systems are available to suspend the solution container. Adjustable freestanding poles may be used, especially for patients who are ambulatory (Figure 8–7). Other poles may attach to chairs, beds, or gurneys. In locations where the IV fluid container will not be moved, devices such as loops or hooks suspended from the ceiling or other suspension systems may be used. The systems used with ambulatory patients also have the ability to be adjusted to place the fluid container at the desired height for the desired flow rate.

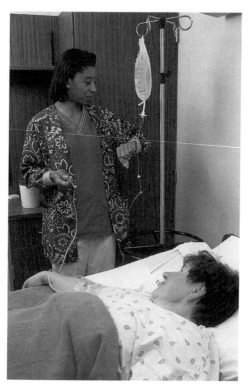

Figure 8-7 Adjustable freestanding IV pole. (From Perry AG, Potter PA: *Clinical nursing skills & techniques,* ed 6, St Louis, 2006, Mosby.)

Supplies for Applying Local Anesthetics Before Venipuncture

Topical medications are available to provide anesthesia to the area of the skin where the venipuncture is to be performed. These medications should be carried to the site for the initiation of the infusion. The exact medication to be used and the route of application are dependent on the preferences of the health care provider or the policies of the place of employment.

Dressing Material and Tape

Dressing materials include sterile gauze, transparent semipermeable membrane dressings, and antimicrobial patches that may be applied under the dressing or used alone. Adequate tape supplies to secure tubing should be available. The medical record should be checked for any possible patient allergies to tape or latex gloves before allowing these to come in contact with the patient's skin. These supplies should also be transported with venipuncture devices and antiseptic wipes. The supplies and equipment are transported to the patient's location. All equipment and supplies should be readily available so the patient does not have to be left during the initiation of the procedure.

PREPARATION OF THE PATIENT

Preparing the patient for IV therapy is similar to patient preparation for any procedure. The technique used to identify the patient may be verbal, asking his or her name, or nonverbal, reading identification bracelets when available. In some inpatient settings, computer identification which compares the patient with the available fluids or medications is used. Whatever the means of patient identification, be sure the correct patient and the correct fluids agree to prevent errors and to increase patient safety.

Explaining the procedure to the patient encourages cooperation and reduces anxiety throughout the process. The explanation may be as simple as showing the patient the correct way to wear the gown and a comfortable position for the therapy. Clarifying that the use of a gown protects personal clothing while allowing access to the arms for the venipuncture should illicit the patient's cooperation. Provide the necessary supplies, such as drapes, for maintenance of modesty and comfort. Finally, answer questions honestly about the procedure to build confidence and trust. Remember, when the patient understands the need for the therapy, the process will be easier for all concerned.

Perform Initial Patient Screening

Preparation of the patient for administration usually involves a baseline screening including a medical history and any known allergies. This screening should include information about the patient's present condition, previous health history issues, and family history. It is prudent to document this information for future reference. A clinical screening including the patient's weight and vital signs is basic.

For those patients who do not require emergency care, crucial elements in prescreening of patients about to receive IV therapy are as follows:

• Temperature
• Pulse
• Respirations
• Blood pressure
• Weight
• Allergies

These measurements provide a baseline for comparison throughout the procedure and after its completion. They also provide an assessment tool for the onset of complications including fluid overload, pulmonary or air emboli, and systemic infection, both during and after the infusion. Some facilities request monitoring intake and output during and immediately after the procedure.

Other observations made during the screening process and the infusion procedure are basic in assessing possibility of fluid imbalance. Signs to assess are as follows:

• Presence of fever
• Presence of perspiration
• Dry, warm skin and cracked lips
• Thirst
• Elasticity of skin
• Absence of moisture in axillae
• Concentrated, dark urine

Any of the signs noted should be documented, as should the vital signs and initial assessment steps.

PREPARATION OF THE EQUIPMENT

Once the physician's order is confirmed, hands are sanitized, equipment is selected and transported to patient area, the patient is identified, and the initial screening is performed, the next step is to assemble the equipment for the initiation of the IV therapy.

Prepare the IV Solution Container for Use

The appropriate solutions must be suspended above the infusion site on the device needed for the type of infusion. When an infusion regulation device is to be used, a pole is required to hold the solution container. The infusion regulation device is attached to the pole and the pole is extended to the proper height for the rate of infusion. When gravity is the force used for infusion, the pole or hanger loop is set at the height to maintain a good flow rate. The clamp on the infusion set will also provide a control of the rate of infusion.

Recheck Medication and Dosage Calculations

Medication and dosage calculations should be rechecked to ensure the proper drug and dose are being administered. Labels for the medications added to fluids will be affixed to the fluid bag (Figure 8–8) so that these can be checked against the orders. Expiration dates are found on all solution containers and sterilized supplies. Solutions may have alterations in composition over a period of time and any outdated solution must never be administered. Outdated supplies may not be sterile and may be contaminated, creating a possibility for infection. Therefore, checking the fluids includes expiration dates, medications, and the actual fluid composition.

Assemble Equipment and Supplies

Equipment and supplies for IV therapy must be carefully handled to prevent contamination; any equipment or supplies that come in direct contact with the IV fluids and infusion site must be kept sterile at all times. These precautions are necessary

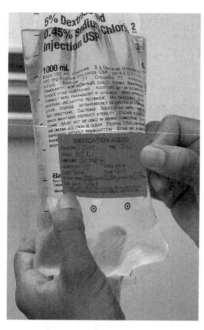

Figure 8-8 Medication label affixed to IV bag. (From Perry AG, Potter PA: *Clinical nursing skills & techniques*, ed 6, St Louis, 2006, Mosby.)

to protect the patient against possible infection. Remember, patient safety is of utmost importance.

- Check the external bag of bagged solutions for any punctures, tears, cuts, or other breach of the integrity of the container. Glass containers should be checked for any cracks in the glass. Both glass containers and bagged solution should be observed for any discoloration, cloudiness, or presence of foreign particles. The presence of any of these factors may be indicative of contamination, and the product must not be used; it should be discarded or returned to the proper source.
- Select the correct administration set and any required filter. When a question arises concerning the proper administration set to be used or if a filter is required, contact the pharmacist for verification of the chosen set and filter.
- Before opening, check the IV solution administration set wrapping for any tears or damage.
- Confirm that the correct solution has been selected. This second confirmation of the

physician's order of the correct solution is necessary for patient safety. This is one of the three befores of medication administration.

- If the solution has been refrigerated, remove it from the refrigerator and allow it to warm slightly. Air bubbles are more easily detected and expelled in a warmer solution.
- Remove the outer wrap from the IV bag and apply gentle pressure to inspect it carefully for any leaks or tears. Hold up the bag and examine it to ascertain any discoloration, cloudiness, or particulate matter that may indicate possible contamination of the fluids. Any breach in the integrity of the solution container indicates possible contamination, and the solution should be discarded if problems are found.
- Mark on the time strip the times when the solution should be infused. Affix the time strip in the proper position to the IV bags, if not done previously.
- Remove tubing from its packaging and close the roller clamp.
- Remove the plastic protector from the tubing spike at the drip chamber end using care to not contaminate the spike. Insert the tubing spike into the bag port while squeezing the drip chamber (Figure 8–9). Once the tubing

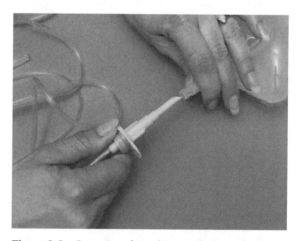

Figure 8-9 Inserting the tubing spike into the bag port. (From Perry AG, Potter PA: *Clinical nursing skills & techniques*, ed 6, St Louis, 2006, Mosby.)

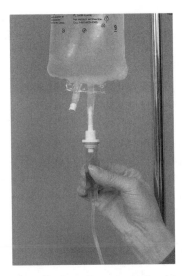

Figure 8-10   Releasing pressure on the drip chamber. (From Perry AG, Potter PA: *Clinical nursing skills & techniques*, ed 6, St Louis, 2006, Mosby.)

spike is inserted into the bag port, release the pressure on the drip chamber, allowing it to partially fill (Figure 8–10). If a terminal filter is required, attach it now.

- Remove the protective cover from the distal end of the tubing, again using care to not contaminate the end. This step may be performed with the container hanging from the suspension system, or it may be accomplished with the container resting on a hard surface. The most important aspect is to remember that all exposed parts of the system must not touch anything to maintain sterility and prevent possible infection.

- Release the roller clamp enough to allow fluid to flow through the tubing, purging the tubing of all air and air bubbles. This step is required to prevent air bubbles from entering the bloodstream with possible consequence of air embolism.

- Invert any "Y" injection sites and tap to purge any residual air from these sites. If a filter is attached, it should be held pointing downward so the portion of the filter closest to the patient fills with fluid first. Then, invert the filter so it can finish filling (priming); tap the filter as it

fills to release any air bubbles that might be trapped.

- When the filter is primed and the tubing has been flushed with fluid removing all air bubbles, close the clamp of the tubing.

- Place a needleless cannula on the end of the tubing to maintain sterility until the system preparation is complete.

- Load the tubing of the administration set into an electronic pump if one is going to be used. Styles of pumps vary in their preparation; directions, including illustrations, are usually attached. Follow the manufacturer's instructions for loading the recommended administration set into the pump delivery mechanism. When a pump system is not going to be used, confirm the times and amounts that are indicated on the marked time strip and ensure that the strip is applied correctly.

Once the equipment preparation is complete, the system is flushed and ready to begin the infusion, the next step is the initiation of IV therapy.

SELECTING A SUITABLE SITE

Site selection includes locating a suitable vein for a venipuncture device to be used and ensuring the size will allow for the volume of fluid to be infused at the rate ordered; considering the type of fluid to be infused, especially the viscosity of the fluid; ensuring patient comfort; and considering possible patient mobility. The location, direction, and condition of the veins should also be considered.

- Begin with examining distal veins, especially those in the hands. It is best to avoid using large veins, keeping them available for emergencies. IVs usually are started in the small veins as close to the hands as possible. Additionally, when more sites are required for subsequent venipunctures, it then is possible to move up the arm to the larger veins closer to the heart without experiencing difficulties from previously injected veins. However, it is not possible to move back distally because the lower veins have been previously used and cannot be used again. Another factor to consider is avoiding veins over sharp bony areas or joints or veins in areas of recent trauma from injury or surgical procedures.

Assess convenient peripheral veins, including the following (from distal to proximal):

- **Back of the hand: Dorsal basilic or cephalic vein (Figure 8–11).** This site permits movement of the arm and allows for ambulation and use of more proximal veins, if necessary.
- **Forearm: Basilic or cephalic vein.** These veins are stable and similar to the veins in the dorsum of the hand, allowing for moving up the arm if a distal site is compromised. This site also permits more mobility for the patient because the site can be easily immobilized to prevent dislocation of the venipuncture device.

- **Antecubital fossa/inner aspect of the elbow: Median basilic and median cephalic vein.** These veins are large, usually visible, readily palpable, and easily accessible. The arm must be immobilized to protect the venipuncture site, to prevent dislocation of the venipuncture device and infiltration of fluids, or both. This site may be uncomfortable for the patient; it is recommended to select a site below the elbow crease for greater patient comfort, and because it is very difficult to locate a site more proximal on the arm when the site is no longer usable.
- **Other available veins: thigh–femoral and great saphenous veins; ankle–great saphenous; foot–dorsal venous arch, or venous plexus of dorsum.** These veins are used as a

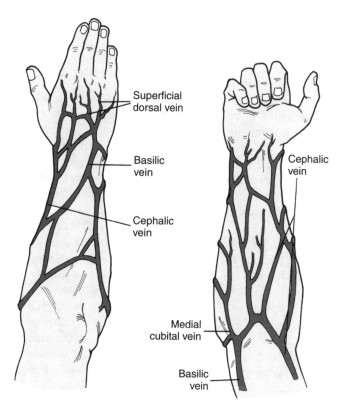

Figure 8-11   Common peripheral IV infusion sites. (From Linton AD, Maebius NK: *Introduction to medical-surgical nursing*, ed 3, Philadelphia, 2003, Saunders.)

last resort and may be difficult to access. The use of these veins usually limits movement of the area and ambulation.

- **Assessing central venous lines.** Clinicians who are specially trained place central venous lines. The procedure for placement of a central line is usually performed under surgical aseptic technique and often as a minor surgical procedure using large peripheral veins (Figure 8–12).

- Scalp veins in the temporal area or veins in the back of the hand or on the dorsum of the foot are commonly used for infants. Special pediatric clinicians usually initiate IV therapy for infants. Small butterflies are used to provide IV fluids to the infant.

Vein Preparation for Venipuncture

Veins require preparation before the venipuncture is attempted. The vein usually must be distended for ease of palpatation and identification prior to insertion of the venipuncture device. Following are methods used to distend veins:

- Apply compression above the site where a needle or catheter is to be inserted.

- When the arm or hand is the site to be used, have the patient clench his or her fist by opening and closing the fist to pump blood into the vessels, causing them to extend.

- Stroke the chosen area to stimulate the flow of blood in the direction of the vein, causing blood to collect and distend the vein.

- Apply a sphygmomanometer cuff on the limb above the intended site, and extend the pressure on the cuff to just below systolic pressure.

- Lightly and gently tap the vein, being careful not to injure the site. Tapping causes the vein to distend, but excessive tapping can result in venous constriction.

- If needed, allow the limb to hang below the level of the body, placing it in a dependent

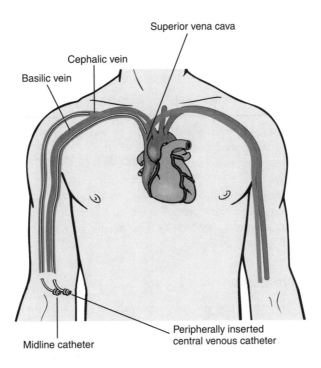

Figure 8-12   A peripherally inserted central catheter. (From Linton AD, Maebius NK: *Introduction to medical-surgical nursing*, ed 3, Philadelphia, 2003, Saunders.)

position for a few minutes to distend the veins with blood. The dependent position allows the pooling of blood in the distal location of the extremity.

- Use a tourniquet or other means of constricting the vein above the intended site to allow blood pooling. Care must be taken that the tourniquet is adequately snug to collect the blood in the veins, but not so tight that arterial blood flow is inhibited.
- Apply moist heat to the area, often with a warm, moist towel to relax the walls of the veins, allowing distention.

Cleansing the Intended Infusion Site

Cleansing antiseptic solutions include 70% isopropyl alcohol, iodophor (iodine preparations), and chlorhexidine gluconate (Hibiclens). When a patient has advised the health care provider of his or her allergy to iodine or alcohol, caution must be used to not expose the patient to either of these products. Chlorhexidine gluconate may be used to cleanse the area as may soap and sterile water if the patient is allergic to other antiseptics.

The procedure for cleansing is performed as follows:

- Cleanse the intended site with the selected antiseptic agent.
- Moving the applicator or gauze in an outward circular motion (from the anticipated site of the venipuncture outward) is the appropriate method of cleansing the area.
- When an iodine and alcohol preparation is used, they should be allowed to dry prior to the insertion of the venipuncture device to prevent a stinging sensation when the skin is broken.

Selection of Venipuncture Device

Factors to consider when selecting the device include the amount of solution to be infused, the type of fluid and its viscosity, and the site of the venipuncture, including the size and condition of the selected vein. Commonly used peripheral infusion insertion devices include over-the-needle catheters, scalp or butterfly needles, and through-the-needle catheters.

Over-the-Needle Catheters

Over-the-needle catheters, the name describing the actual components of the device, may be found with just the hub of the needle or with wings for ease of insertion. During venipuncture, the needle point or stylet at the distal tip is used for the insertion of the peripheral device through the skin and into the vein. When the catheter enters the vein, blood flashes back into the hub and the catheter is threaded off the stylet into the vein, followed by the stylet (the sharp metal probe used to puncture the skin and into the vein) being removed and discarded. The flexible catheter is left within the vein for the infusion of fluids. These catheters range from $1/2$ inch to 2 inches in length and are in even-number gauges. Following are the usual sizes and uses of over-the-needle catheters:

- Gauges from 14 to 18 are used for major surgery, trauma, or blood administration.
- 20 gauge is most often used with adults.
- 22-gauge devices are appropriate for pediatric patients and adults with small veins.

These devices are inserted much like a needle and provide a patency for a longer period of time without the potential of additional trauma to the vein by a needle point.

Scalp Vein or Butterfly Needles

Frequently used for short-term therapy, scalp vein or butterfly needles are excellent for one-time medication administration intravenously. The needle attaches easily to the tubing. Needle sizes are in odd-number gauges from 17 to 25 with the length varying from $1/2$ inch to 1 inch. The butterfly needle has plastic wings attached to the hub and tubing that extends 3 to 12 inches past the needle with the hub for connection. Made of stainless steel, there is the possibility of accidental puncturing of the vein walls, increasing the risk for infiltration. This type of infusion device should not be used at a site in which movement is anticipated. Butterfly needles are often used with infants, small children, and the elderly for venipuncture because they have small and fragile veins.

Through-the-Needle Catheters

The least commonly used venipuncture device is the through-the-needle catheter, in which the catheter is found within the lumen of the needle. The needle is used for the insertion of the catheter and then withdrawn and secured on the outside of the skin. Sizes include 14- to 19-gauge needles surrounding the catheter. The length of the needle ranges from 1 inch to 2 inches, and the catheter's length ranges from 8 to 36 inches. Viscous fluids and drugs are administered through these relatively stable devices.

STEPS IN THE INITIATION OF IV INFUSION THERAPY

Preparation Prior to Venipuncture

Steps for preparing the patient and equipment for the initiation of an infusion in the upper limb follow:
- Step 1: Confirm the physician's order.
- Step 2: Sanitize hands.
- Step 3: Confirm the patient's identity.
- Step 4: Explain the procedure to the patient and answer any questions concerning the process.
- Step 5: Perform prescreening procedures and document vital signs, any reported allergies, and any observations of the patient's condition.
- Step 6: Prepare cleansing applicators, dressing material, and tape to be readily available and within reach for use at the time of the venipuncture.
- Step 7: Place IV solution container with attached administration set on a pole or suspension device.
- Step 8: Make the patient comfortable, usually in a semireclining or reclining position. Ensure the arm being used is removed from patient clothing or the patient has on a gown so the vein site can be easily palpated and accessed.

- Step 9: Examine the area where the venipuncture is to be done. When possible, select the nondominant limb and a vein that is in the distal portion of that limb. Veins should be as straight as possible and not over bony parts. Palpate for arteries and if necessary use a mini ultrasound device to locate arteries and, if possible, nearby nerves. Determine the size of the vein is appropriate for the type of fluid to be infused and the rate of infusion ordered. Select a large, visible vein if at all possible. The vein should dilate easily when held below the body. Consider the comfort of the patient and needs for ambulation. The skin and tissue surrounding the intended site should also be assessed for fragility.
- Step 10: Place the tourniquet or other device for compression under the arm above the intended venipuncture site (lower arm for veins in the hand), and ensure the hand or arm is supported to hold it in place. Often, the hand is held in the clinician's nondominant hand for ease of movement as needed by the clinician.
- Step 11: The prepared IV administration set's terminal end is placed on a sterile field (or covered to ensure sterility) for easy access by the clinician. (The set has been flushed with solution and a sterile cap has been placed on the terminal aspect of the tubing.)
- Step 12: The site has been selected and a possible venipuncture device is selected and set within reach of the clinician. Other butterflies and catheters should also be available in close proximity.

Venipuncture Procedure

With the preparation concluded, progressing on to the venipuncture is described as follows:
- Step 1: Apply tourniquet or other compression device 3 to 6 inches above proposed venipuncture site. A slip-knot is used on the tourniquet for easy release (Figure 8–13). Check for radial pulse to confirm that blood flow to the distal areas has not been compromised by a tourniquet that is too tight. If the tourniquet

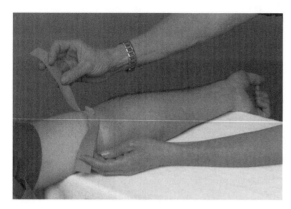

Figure 8-13 Placement of tourniquet. (From Perry AG, Potter PA: *Clinical nursing skills & techniques,* ed 6, St Louis, 2006, Mosby.)

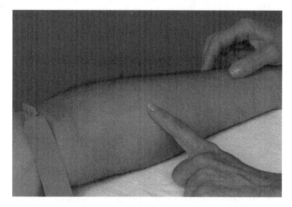

Figure 8-14 Palpate vein. (From Perry AG, Potter PA: *Clinical nursing skills & techniques,* ed 6, St Louis, 2006, Mosby.)

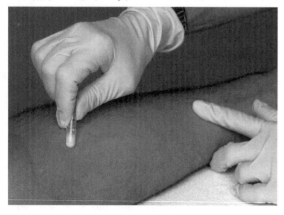

Figure 8-15 Cleanse the site. (From Perry AG, Potter PA: *Clinical nursing skills & techniques,* ed 6, St Louis, 2006, Mosby.)

is in place for more than 2 minutes, it should be released and blood is allowed to flow into the area.

- Step 2: Palpate the selected vein with fingertips (Figure 8–14).
- Step 3: Don gloves and other personal protective equipment following Occupational Safety and Health Administration (OSHA) guidelines for barrier protection as appropriate.
- Step 4: Cleanse the site with appropriate antiseptic wipes using a circular pattern moving from the chosen puncture site to the outside. Allow skin to air dry (Figure 8–15).
- Step 5: Ask the patient to open and close his or her fist several times to distend veins.
- Step 6: Hold the venipuncture device in the dominant hand while stretching the skin of the proposed site with the other hand, stabilizing the vein (Figure 8–16).
- Step 7: Hold the needle at a 10- to 30-degree angle alongside the vein with the bevel up. The angle of the needle depends on the depth of the vein in the tissue.
- Step 8: Tell the patient that a sharp, quick stick will occur. Pierce the skin by inserting the needle distal and parallel to the vein at a 10- to 30-degree angle to the skin (Figure 8–17). Once the vein is entered, blood will flow back into the tubing or catheter hub.
- Step 9: Release the tension on the skin and slowly advance the needle into the vein approximately 1 inch (Figure 8–18).
- Step 10: Stabilize the needle or catheter with one hand and slowly release the tourniquet with the other hand. If the catheter is used, cover the stylet with the safety cap as it is removed. Keep the needle stable and dispose of the stylet in a rigid biohazard container.
- Step 11: Remove the cap on the end of the tubing and connect the tubing to the hub of the needle or catheter (Figure 8–19).
- Step 12: Slowly release the clamp on the administration set tubing, allowing the solution to flow into the vein. Set the clamp for the desired rate. When a pump is being used, engage the pump to run and set at the appropriate rate of administration in drops per minute or

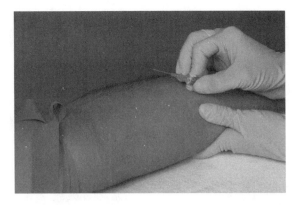

Figure 8-16   Stabilize the vein with nondominant hand; use venipuncture device in dominant hand. (From Perry AG, Potter PA: *Clinical nursing skills & techniques,* ed 6, St Louis, 2006, Mosby.)

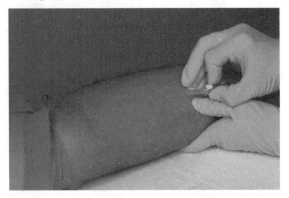

Figure 8-17   Puncture skin with venipuncture device. (From Perry AG, Potter PA: *Clinical nursing skills & techniques,* ed 6, St Louis, 2006, Mosby.)

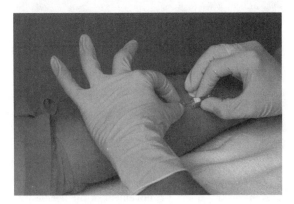

Figure 8-18   Advance venipuncture device into vein. (From Perry AG, Potter PA: *Clinical nursing skills & techniques,* ed 6, St Louis, 2006, Mosby.)

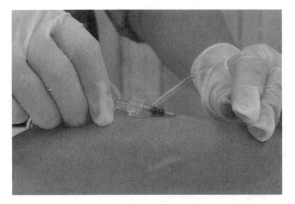

Figure 8-19   Connect end of tubing. (From Perry AG, Potter PA: *Clinical nursing skills & techniques,* ed 6, St Louis, 2006, Mosby.)

milliliters per hour depending on the calibration of the equipment.

- Step 13: Cleanse the skin of any unintentional blood from the skin or tubing.
- Step 14: Remove gloves and dispose of these appropriately in the biohazard waste container, depending on the degree of contamination.
- Step 15: Apply dressing over the site using sterile supplies, either sterile gauze or a sterile semipermeable occlusive dressing (Figure 8–20). The gauze dressing will prevent visualization of the venipuncture site and it may have to be

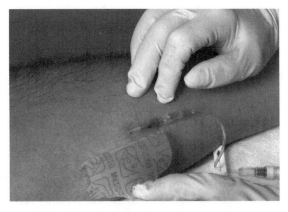

Figure 8-20   Semipermeable occlusive application. (From Perry AG, Potter PA: *Clinical nursing skills & techniques,* ed 6, St Louis, 2006, Mosby.)

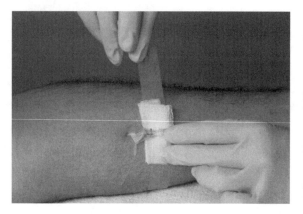

Figure 8-21 Place folded gauze under cannula hub for comfort and safety of patient.

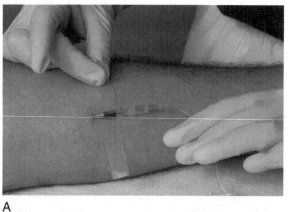

A

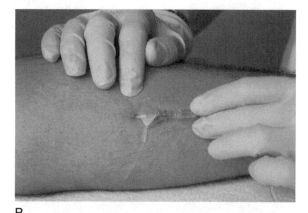

B

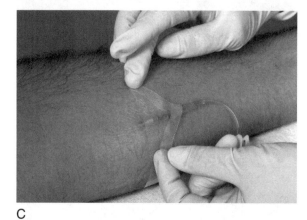

C

Figure 8-22 **A,** Tape is placed under catheter hub. **B,** Chevron is applied. **C,** Chevron tape applied to prevent dislodgement or movement of the needle. (From Perry AG, Potter PA: *Clinical nursing skills & techniques,* ed 6, St Louis, 2006, Mosby.)

lifted to observe the actual venipuncture site. The occlusive dressing allows for visualization of the site and is generally the dressing of choice. Regardless of the type of dressing, a small piece of folded gauze should be placed between the hub of the needle and the skin to prevent pressure and pain (Figure 8–21). The hub should then be secured with a chevron of tape to prevent movement or dislodgment (Figure 8–22). If a butterfly is used, the wings should be taped to the skin and a sterile dressing should be applied over the entire butterfly needle.

- Step 16: Anchor tubing with an adhesive-type tape. Some facilities require time and date of insertion to be marked on the tape along with the clinician's initials (Figure 8–23).
- Step 17: Once again, check and adjust the flow rate of the solution as needed. Check the venipuncture site for any bleeding or leakage of fluid. Make adjustments as needed.
- Step 18: Assure that the patient is in a comfortable position and has a means of calling for assistance should it be necessary.
- Step 19: Document the procedure including the type and amount of solution, the type of needle or catheter used, the location of the venipuncture site, the flow rate of the

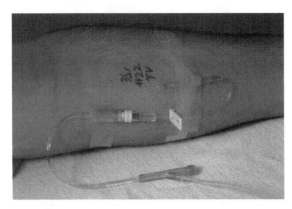

Figure 8-23   Label IV dressing. (From Perry AG, Potter PA: *Clinical nursing skills & techniques,* ed 6, St Louis, 2006, Mosby.)

solution, and how the patient tolerated the procedure.

• Step 20: Dispose of any contaminated waste material or personal protective equipment according to OSHA guidelines.

CARE, ASSESSMENT, AND MAINTENANCE OF THE INFUSION SITE

Regular checks (at least hourly) should be made on the patient receiving IV therapy.

• The venipuncture site should be observed several times in the first 30 minutes and then at least hourly. The observation should include any signs of infiltration, leakage, bleeding, or potential infection. Refer to Chapter 6 for additional information. Should the patient express feeling wetness around the dressing or pain or tightness near the venipuncture site, the complaint should be immediately investigated by the clinician. Redness or abnormal warmth around the site should be noted, and appropriate corrective measures should be taken. When infiltration is suspected and there is no blood return in the tubing when the container is lowered below the infusion site, the IV should be discontinued and restarted at a

different location. Any other possible complications at the site should be addressed as described in Chapter 6.

Important Steps for Maintenance of IV Infusion

• It is imperative that the flow rate be monitored at least hourly after the first 30 minutes of infusion. Rates may be slowed when it is noticed that too much fluid has infused; however, **flow rates should never be increased to make up for flow rates that have slowed.**
• Intake and output records should be maintained while the patient is receiving IV therapy.
• Vital signs should be monitored on a regular basis and documented. Any sudden change of any of the vital signs may be indicative of a systemic reaction to the IV therapy. A complete evaluation of the situation is required, including reporting the findings to the physician.

REPLACEMENT OF THE ORDERED FLUIDS AND MEDICATIONS

IV fluids are often used for replacement therapy and for the delivery of certain medications. However, when large amounts of fluid are not required or desired, two other methods may be used to administer medications: IV piggyback (IVPB) and IV bolus. A third option is a **saline** or **heparin lock.**

IVPB Medication Administration

The piggyback addition to an IV is a method to introduce medication into the patient's bloodstream without disrupting the established IV infusion (Figure 8–24). The secondary administration set as described in Chapter 4 is assembled, and the container (usually a bag of fluid—50 to 250 cc) is hung from the suspension system. The drip chamber is filled half way and the tubing is purged of air by allowing the fluid to run through in the same manner as a primary IV line. The main fluid container is lowered with a hook

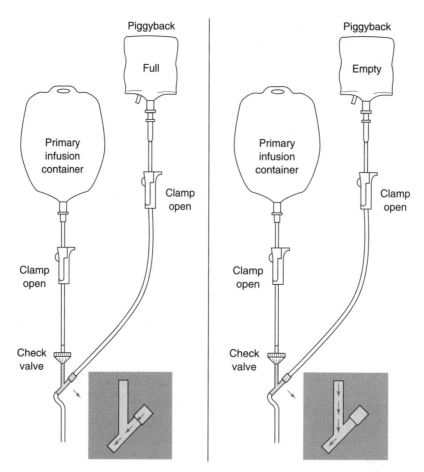

Figure 8-24 Piggyback intermittent administration setup. (From Clayton BD, Stock YN: *Basic pharmacology for nurses*, ed 13, St Louis, 2004, Mosby.)

making it lower than the secondary solution container. Once this is in position, the secondary set tubing is connected to a port on the primary tubing after the port has been cleansed with an antiseptic preparation. The flow control clamp to the secondary set is opened and the primary flow automatically stops, allowing the IVPB fluid to flow into the main IV line. When all the fluid from the piggyback is infused, the mainline IV will again continue its infusion because the back-check value automatically opens when the IVPB fluid falls below the level of the primary line. Piggyback administration is a common method used to deliver antibiotics on an intermittent basis.

Bolus Administration of IV Medication

IV medications ordered to be administered by the "IV push" or bolus method must be administered with great care. Once a medication is pushed into the vein it cannot be retrieved. An additional consideration is the risk of infection when the IV port or cannula hub is entered to administer the medication. The time indicated for administration must be closely followed and the patient must be observed constantly throughout the administration of medication in this manner. Before administering a bolus of medication, the infusion site should be checked for placement within the vein. In addition, the person administering the medication must check the dilution and any possible adverse reactions. Be continuously aware that the the concentration of medication directly into the vein requires special aseptic technique with a professional knowledge to ensure patient safety.

Administering Saline or Heparin IV

The saline lock or heparin lock is used when intermittent IV medications are to be administered. Venipuncture is performed as previously described; however, instead of attaching the IV administration set tubing, an adapter is attached. This port is filled with either normal saline or heparin and it must be flushed before any medication is pushed through it. The adapter or port is secured to the skin around the site and is available for either an IV bolus injection or a piggyback drug administration.

These measures or avenues provide the clinician other means of providing the patient with drug and IV therapy (as ordered by the physician) than just the primary IV lines.

DISCONTINUATION OF IV THERAPY

Once the prescribed infusion is complete, it may be discontinued if the site will not be used for more fluids in the future when the fluids have infiltrated, adverse conditions have occurred, or the vein has been used longer than is acceptable by the policy of the facility. The procedure of discontinuing the IV and removing the venipuncture device should be explained to the patient. Any patient concerns or questions must be addressed in a tactful and trusting manner to gain the necessary cooperation.

To discontinue the fluids, the following steps are needed:

- The tubing is clamped shut, and the infusion device is turned off, if applicable.
- The clinician loosens any tape and applies gloves.
- A gauze pad is held in the nondominant hand to be used to apply gentle pressure over the site as the needle or catheter is removed.
- The needle or catheter is gripped by the dominant hand and slowly withdrawn following the pathway of the vein (Figure 8–25).

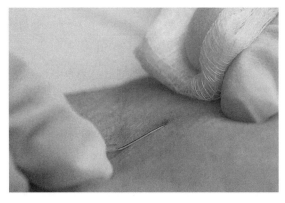

Figure 8-25   Withdraw IV catheter. (From Perry AG, Potter PA: *Clinical nursing skills & techniques,* ed 6, St Louis, 2006, Mosby.)

- Pressure is held on the site until bleeding ceases.
- A sterile dressing is applied to the site (often, a pressure dressing is required to apply gentle pressure over the site) and taped in place.
- The patient is assessed for how the procedure was tolerated.
- The discontinuation of the therapy is documented including date, time, total amount and type of fluid infused, assessment of appearance of site, any significant observations of the patient, and name or initials of clinician discontinuing the IV infusion.
- All contaminated and used supplies and equipment are discarded according to OSHA guidelines with any sharps being placed in sharps containers and other materials properly disposed in the correct waste containers.
- The patient is assisted to the area of dismissal, as appropriate.

The policy of the site of employment may vary slightly from the steps given in this text, but need for patient safety using appropriate aseptic technique is always the goal of IV therapy. As IV therapy continues to be a more prevalent procedure in both inpatient and ambulatory care for routine and specialized care, the clinician must be entirely aware of the correct procedure for safe patient care.

REVIEW QUESTIONS

1. What are the important aspects of the physician's order to be checked prior to initiating IV therapy?

2. List observations of the patient that should be made throughout both the screening process and the infusion procedure that are basic in assessing possibility of fluid imbalance.

3. Explain the rationale for purging the administration set of air bubbles.

4. What are the two main types of IV drip chambers found in IV administration sets?

5. What are major factors to consider when selecting a vein for an infusion site?

6. Identify methods used to distend veins preparing for the venipuncture.

7. Explain the actual venipuncture.

8. Discuss observation of the infusions site as to frequency of observations and nature of observations.

9. In addition to infusion of fluids, what other types of IV administration are available?

10. What are the steps to be taken when discontinuing an IV?

A
IV Drug Solution Compatibility Chart

	D₅	D₁₀	D₅		NS	R	LR	OTHER
			½S	S				
Acetazolamide	C	C	C	C	C	C	C	
Acyclovir	C							
Alpha₁-proteinase inhibitor								Sterile water for inj
Alprostadil	C	C			C			
Alteplase								Sterile water for inj
Amdinocillin	C	C	C	C	C	C	C	D₅ in R
Amikacin	C				C			
Aminocaproic acid			C	C	C	C		D in distilled water
Ammonium Cl					C			May add KCl to solution
Amphotericin B	C							
Ampicillin	C				C			
Amrinone lactate					C			0.45% saline
Antithrombin III	C				C			Sterile water for inj
Ascorbic acid	C				C	C	C	Sodium lactate
Atenolol	C				C			0.45% saline
Azlocillin	C		C		C			
Aztreonam	C	C			C	C	C	Normosol-R
Bretylium tosylate	C				C			
Cefamandole	C				C			
Cefazolin	C				C			
Cefotetan	C				C			
Cefoxitin	C	C			C	C	C	Aminosol
Ceftrazidime	C		C	C	C	C	C	M/G sodium lactate
Ceftriaxone	C				C			
Cefuroxime	C		C	C		C		M/G sodium lactate
Cephalothin	C				C	C	C	M/G sodium lactate
Cephapirin	C				C			
Ciprofloxacin	C				C			
Cyclosporine	C				C			Use only glass containers
Dobutamine					C			Sodium lactate
Dopamine	C		C	C	C		C	M/G sodium lactate
Doxycycline	C				C			Invert sugar 10%
Edetate Na	C	C						Isotonic saline
Ganciclovir	C				C	C	C	
Gentamicin	C				C			Normosol-R

Continued

| | D5 | D10 | D5 | | NS | R | LR | OTHER |
			1/2S	S				
Heparin Na	C	C			C	C		
Ifosfamide	C				C		C	Sterile water for inj
Isoproterenol	C			C	C	C		Invert sugar 5% & 10%
Kanamycin	C				C			
Metaraminol	C			C	C	C	C	Normosol-R
Methicillin	C			C				
Metoclopramide	C			C		C	C	
Mezlocillin	C	C	C	C	C	C	C	Fructose 5%
Moxalactam	C	C	C	C	C	C	C	M/G sodium lactate
Netilmicin	C	C		C	C	C	C	Normosol-R
Nitroglycerin	C	C			C			
Norepinephrine	C	C		C			C	
Piperacillin	C			C	C		C	
Ritodrine	C							
Ticarcillin	C				C		C	
Tobramycin	C				C			
Vidarabine	C	C			C			

This chart is not inclusive and is based on manufacturers' recommendations.

Key

C = Compatible

D5 = Dextrose 5%

D10 = Dextrose 10%

D5 1/2S = Dextrose 5% in saline 0.45%

D5S = Dextrose 5% in saline 0.9%

NS = Sodium chloride 0.9% (normal saline)

R = Ringer's solution

LR = Lactated Ringer's solution

(From Skidmore-Roth L: Mosby's Drug Guide for Nurses, 7 ed, Mosby, 2006, St Louis.)

Assemble and Prepare Equipment, Supplies, and the Patient for IV Infusion

Student Name: _____   Date: _____

TASK: To assemble the necessary equipment, supplies, and the patient for an IV infusion

CONDITIONS: Given the proper information from the physician's order in the medical record, the student will be able to assemble the following equipment and supplies for IV infusion using appropriate quality controls.

EQUIPMENT AND SUPPLIES
- Fluids, as ordered by health care professional
- Correct administration set to provide fluids at flow rate ordered
- Alcohol swabs
- Bandaging supplies
- Tourniquet
- Local anesthetic, if appropriate
- Pen
- IV pole or other mounting for the fluids
- Volume control device, such as pump, as appropriate
- Waste container
- Patient gown, as indicated

STANDARDS: Complete the competency, achieving 100% accuracy of all steps in two attempts or standards at the discretion of the evaluator.

Steps	1st Attempt	2nd Attempt
1. Check the physician's orders and confirm the identity of the patient.		
2. Review of patient's history for indications that affect IV therapy.		

Continued

Steps	1st Attempt	2nd Attempt

3. Sanitize hands appropriately.

4. Assemble supplies starting with correct solution in the designated volume, as appropriate for order.

5. Select or verify that the correct administration set and tubing to supply fluids at ordered flow rate is available including extensions for tubing if indicated.

6. Assemble antiseptic solutions and applicators.

7. Assemble venipuncture/infusion devices that are appropriate for the physician's orders.

8. Assemble devices for regulation and evaluation of fluid flow, such as appropriate infusion device or pump, clamps on tubing or measurement tapes for marking flow rates.

9. Select appropriate device for holding solution container, such as an IV pole.

10. Assemble supplies for applying local anesthetics prior to venipuncture if appropriate.

11. Select and assemble dressing material, including sterile bandaging supplies and transparent dressings as indicated.

12. Transport supplies and equipment to the patient's location.

13. Identify the patient and supply clothing.

14. Perform initial screening of the patient, using the medical record for information and then observe patient for past history, signs and symptoms that might affect the fluid infusion. Document findings as appropriate.

15. Explain the procedure to the patient and provide appropriate clothing for the infusion (such as gown with snaps on the shoulder) as necessary.

16. Assist the patient into a gown if necessary and make comfortable on the examination table or bed as appropriate.

17. Prepare the IV fluid container using the steps below:
    a. Recheck dosage calculations and expiration dates on all equipment and supplies.
    b. Check the external bag of solution for any punctures or cuts (examine glass containers for any cracks). Observe containers for any discoloration, cloudiness or presence of foreign particles in the fluids. Check IV administration set wrapping for any tears or damage before opening. Remove any refrigerated solution from the refrigerator in adequate time to allow it to warm prior to administration.

Steps	1st Attempt	2nd Attempt

c. Confirm that the correct solution has been selected by checking before taking from storage, before preparing for infusion, and before taking to the patient room. Also be sure to use the 7 "Rights" of medication administration.

d. Again, reevaluate the selection of the correct administration set with any required filter.

e. Remove the outer wrap from the IV bag and apply gentle pressure while inspecting for any leaks or tears. Discard fluids if there seems to be a break in quality control.

f. If a time strip is used for infusion, mark the time strip with the times for the solution infusion and place the label on the bag.

g. Remove tubing from its packaging and close the roller clamp.

h. Remove the plastic protector from the tubing spike at drip chamber end, using care to not contaminate the spike. Insert the tubing spike into the bag port while squeezing the drip chamber.

i. When tubing spike is inserted into the bag port, release the pressure on the drip chamber allowing it to partially fill. If terminal filter is required, attach now.

j. Remove the protective cover from the distal end of the tubing, again using care to not contaminate the tubing end.

18. Release the roller clamp to allow fluid to flow through tubing to purge tubing of all air including bubbles. Tap tubing, as necesssary, to remove any remaining bubbles.

19. Invert "Y" injection sites and tap to purge residual air from these sites.

20. When the tubing has been purged of air, place a needleless cannula on the end of tubing to maintain sterility until set-up is complete.

21. Load fluids into an electronic pump if appropriate and check pump for proper functioning.

22. Dispose of nonbiohazard waste as appropriate.

23. Once preparation of equipment is complete, system is flushed by allowing 5 ml of fluid to run through the tubing. The next step in the initiation of IV therapy. (See competency sheet for initiating IV therapy.)

Evaluator's Signature: _____

1st Attempt Grade: _____
2nd Attempt Grade: _____

Evaluator's Possible Points
1st Attempt Points: _____
2nd Attempt Points: _____

Initiating IV Therapy

Student Name: _____   Date: _____

TASK: Initiate an IV infusion

CONDITIONS: Given the proper information from the physician's order in the medical record and the prepared supplies and equipment, the student will be able to prepare a site for and initiate IV therapy.

EQUIPMENT AND SUPPLIES
- Fluids, as prepared in previous competency
- Alcohol swabs
- Bandaging supplies
- Tourniquet
- Anesthetic, if appropriate
- Pen
- IV pole or other mounting for the fluids
- Clamp or volume control device
- Disposable gloves
- Sharps container
- Waste container

STANDARDS: Complete the competency, achieving 100% accuracy of all steps in two attempts or standards at the discretion of the evaluator.

Steps	1st Attempt	2nd Attempt
1. Sanitize hands.*		
2. Assemble equipment, solution and supplies as prepared during the competency for assembling supplies for IV therapy.*		
3. Confirm patient's identity.*		
4. Explain procedure to patient, answering any questions.*		
5. Perform prescreening procedures. Document vital signs, reported allergies, and observations.*		
6. Place prepared IV solution container on suspension device.*		
7. Place patient in a comfortable position, with arm for infusion removed from clothing or placed in a gown that allows easy access over a period of time.*		

* Steps may have been completed previously if the preparation of fluids has been accomplished just prior to the infusion procedure.

Steps	1st Attempt	2nd Attempt

8. Place cleansing applicators, dressing material, and tape within reach.

9. Confirm physician's order to the solution being infused.

10. Examine the site for venipuncture to find an appropriate vein for infusion. Assess skin and tissue surrounding the intended site for integrity.

11. Place tourniquet or other device for compression under the arm above the intended venipuncture site.

12. Place IV administration set terminal on a sterile field with venipuncture device within reach. Have other venipuncture devices of various sizes available at close proximity for use, if necessary. If the cover for the administration device has been removed, a sterile fluid must be used.

13. Don personal protective equipment following OSHA guidelines. Note: Gloves may be donned following the palpation of the vein but must be applied prior to preparing the site for venipuncture.

14. Apply tourniquet or other compression device 3–6 inches above proposed venipuncture site. Check for radial pulse to confirm that arterial blood flow has not been compromised by tourniquet application that is too tight.

15. Select a vein, (preferably the nondominant limb with a vein in the distal portion). Palpate selected vein with finger tips. Be sure the vein is sufficiently large to allow placement of the selected device, such as a catheter or needle.

16. Cleanse site with appropriate antiseptic wipes using circular pattern from the inside to the outside. Allow skin to air dry.

17. Ask patient to open and close fist several times to distend veins.

18. Remove the cover for the venipuncture device and with the venipuncture device in dominant hand, use the thumb of nondominant hand below the vein to stretch the skin of proposed site to stabilize vein.

19. Hold the needle at a 45° angle along vein with the bevel up.

20. Advise the patient that a sharp, quick stick will occur. Pierce skin by inserting needle distal and parallel to the vein at a 10 to 30° angle to skin. Watch for blood backflow into tubing or catheter hub.

21. Slowly advance needle into the vein approximately one inch and release tension on skin. Lower needle so almost flush with skin.

Continued

Steps	1ˢᵗ Attempt	2ⁿᵈ Attempt

22. Stabilize needle or catheter using dominant hand and slowly release tourniquet If catheter used, remove safety cap from stylet and dispose of in rigid biohazard container.

23. Remove cap on end of tubing and quickly connect tubing to hub of needle or catheter without touching the point of entry of the adapter.

24. Slowly release clamp on tubing allowing the solution to flow into vein. Set for desired rate if clamp is used. If using pump, engage to run and set at appropriate rate of administration.

25. Gently cleanse skin and tubing of any unintentional blood or other fluids and properly dispose of the cleansing supplies. Check fluids to be sure that no leaking of fluids or blood is present.

26. Remove gloves and dispose in appropriate waste container.

27. Apply sterile dressing at the site. Place a small piece of folded gauze between the hub of the needle and the skin to prevent pressure and pain. Secure hub with chevron of tape placed around the hub and then attached near the site to prevent movement or dislodgment. Do **not** cover the hub with tape. If butterfly infusion set is used, tape wings of the device to the skin and cover entirely with sterile dressing.

28. Loop the tubing along the arm and anchor tubing with tape, marking the tape with time and date of insertion, size and length of needle or catheter, and initials of person performing procedure.

29. Recheck and adjust flow rate of the solution as needed. Again inspect venipuncture site for bleeding or leakage of fluid and swelling along the venipuncture site.

30. Check patient for comfortable position and means to call for assistance as necessary.

31. Document procedure including type and amount of solution, type of needle or catheter, location of venipuncture site, flow rate, and how patient tolerated the procedure.

32. Dispose of any contaminated waste material or personal protective equipment according to OSHA guidelines.

Evaluator's Signature: _____

1st Attempt Grade: _____

2nd Attempt Grade: _____

Evaluator's Possible Points

1st Attempt Points: _____

2nd Attempt Points: _____

C
Answers to Review Questions

CHAPTER 1

1. The type of fluids ordered for the patient depends on the patient's state of homeostasis and/or the need for nutrition.
2. The goals of IV therapy are to maintain or restore normal fluid volume and electrolyte balance for homeostasis and to provide a means of quickly and efficiently administering medications.
3. For a medication to be effective, the medication must reach the blood stream for distribution throughout the body. With oral and other parenteral medications, the drug must be absorbed and must cross barriers such as those in the tissues and the digestive tract. With the IV administration, the medication is administered directly into the blood stream and these barriers do not exist.
4. Medications are given intravenously when the medication might be detrimental to tissues because the IV route prevents tissue damage by the exposure to the medication with proper administration into the veins.
5. The three rationales for IV therapy are maintenance therapy, replacement therapy, and restoration therapy.
6. Cultural and ethnic beliefs are important because these are the basis for one's perceptions, judgments, behavior, and self-understanding. These beliefs are the basis for how the person reacts to IV therapy.
7. The role of the person administering intravenous therapy is limited by the medical practices act of the state of practice but the competency level of the procedure to be performed and the educational background of the person performing the competency also must be considered prior to administering intravenous therapy.
8. Standard of care is that care which is expected in the circumstance in which it is given and that a professional is providing the care that a typical person with the knowledge and skill base would provide in the same circumstances. This care must be typical of the care given in the same geographic area.
9. Negligence occurs when the person administering IV medications or fluids does not act in a reasonable and prudent manner. Malpractice is when the professional has departed from the standards of care health care professional with the same level of professional knowledge would provide in similar circumstances.
10. Each person is liable for the actions they take with IV therapy, including the physician who orders the therapy, the professional who initiates the therapy, and the person monitoring the patient throughout the administration.

CHAPTER 2

1. Homeostasis is defined as the relative constancy of internal environment of the human body that is maintained by adaptive responses to promote health and survival. The steady state is maintained through feedback as well as various sensual mechanisms that provide organs with the needed responses to maintain

this internal balance essential for survival. Balance of the body's internal environment includes balancing of body fluids and chemical substances, some of which include electrolytes, that are dissolved in the fluids. The dynamic equilibrium between the fluids and electrolytes involves a delicate balance to maintain homeostasis that supports processes necessary to maintain life.

2. Blood returns to the right upper chamber of the heart (atrium) via the superior and inferior vena cava. From the right atrium blood is pumped through the tricuspid or AV valve to the right ventricle. Blood then is pumped from the right ventricle through the pulmonic valves into the pulmonary arteries and then on to the lungs for pulmonary circulation. Blood leaves the lungs via the pulmonary veins and is transported back to the left upper chamber of the heart, the left atrium. It travels through the mitral or bicuspid valve into the left lower chamber, the left ventricle. The blood is then pumped through the aortic valve into the aorta to be returned to systemic circulation.

3. Arteries carry oxygenated blood away from the heart; except the pulmonary arteries, which are the only arteries of the body that carry oxygen-poor blood. Veins return deoxygenated blood to the heart; except the pulmonary veins, which are the only veins that carry oxygen rich blood.

4. Capillaries are very minute vessels in the circulatory system that connect arterioles and venules. Their walls are one cell think allowing for easy passage of fluids, nutrients, gases and some solutes into and out of tissue.

5. The walls of veins, like the walls of arteries consist of three concentric layers, the tunica interna, the tunica media and the tunica externa. In arteries, there is less smooth muscle and connective tissue, making them thinner and less rigid. Veins have a tendency to collapse when not under pressure or distended by blood. Medium to large veins often contain valves to keep the blood flowing toward the heart.

6. Veins often contain valves to keep the blood flowing toward the heart and to prevent from causing a reverse in the flow of blood back to the capillaries. Blood pressure in veins normally is low and it is not able to oppose the force of gravity. The valves located in the tunica interna permit the blood to flow in one direction, toward the heart and prevent any backward flow back into the capillaries.

7. Blood as the liquid tissue in the body, provides the transport medium necessary to support life through nutrition to tissues and excretion of waste products. In addition to the activity of transporting essential elements required to support life, blood also is involved in regulation activities as well as in protection of the body. The transportation activity includes nutrients and oxygen to the cells, hormones to target tissues, carbon dioxide to the lungs and other waste products of cellular metabolism to the kidneys for elimination. It also is involved in regulation of body temperature, fluid and electrolyte balance and in balance of the pH of the body. As a source of protection for the body, blood plays an active role during the clotting process when fluid is leaking from damaged tissue. Additionally, specific white blood cells, phagocytes, target invading microorganisms to prevent infection and disease. Other cells in the blood plasma, antibodies, also help to fend off disease as they react to antigens found with invading microorganisms.

8. Osmosis occurs when solvent molecules move through a selectively permeable membrane from an area where there is a higher concentration of molecules into an area where there is an area of lower concentration of molecules. The process is complete when equilibrium is reached and the solution on both sides of the membrane has the same concentration of solutes.

9. There are three states of concentration of solutes in body fluids. There are three main types of fluids: isotonic fluids, hypotonic fluids and hypertonic fluids. Isotonic fluids are when the solutes in the fluids constitute a neutral

state or the state of solutes normally found in the body. Hypotonic is when the concentration of solutes is lower than normal body state. Hypertonic is the state that occurs when the solutes are in greater concentration that normal body fluids. When hypotonic or hypertonic fluid concentrates are used for replacement, it is possible that body cells will be destroyed as the cells either shrivel up due to loss of water (crenate) or the opposite when they take up water and swell and the cell membrane rupture (lysis). When the rupture occurs in a red blood cell it is termed hemolysis.

10. The fluid contained within the cell walls is referred to as intracellular fluid; that which is outside the cell wall is extracellular fluid. The extracellular fluid is found in the interstitial space. Intracellular and extracellular fluids move across the cell walls by diffusion, osmosis and filtration. During the process of diffusion, particles or molecules move from and area of higher concentration fluids to an area of lower concentration until equal distribution in the fluid is achieved. During the process of osmosis, there is a passage of solvent through semi-permeable membrane that separates different concentrations. Movement is from an area of higher concentration of water molecules into an area of lower concentration of water molecules.

CHAPTER 3

1. Asepsis is the absence of pathogens to provide an environment that is pathogen free. Contamination is when items and the environment are soiled, unclean and no longer sterile.
2. Proper and frequent hand washing or hand hygiene.
3. Disinfectants kill the microorganisms and are used on inanimate objects or surfaces. They are not to be used on skin. Antispetics interfere with cellular metabolism and replication of microorganisms usually resulting in the death of the microorganism. They can be used on skin.

4. Full strength household bleach, phenol, and formaldehyde.
5. 70% isopropyl alcohol, iodine preparations and chlorhexidine gluconate.
6. • The reservoir host (source)
   • A means of exit from the host (portal of exit from the host)
   • A means or method of transmission from the first host to the next host
   • The means of entrance into the next host (portal of entry into the susceptible host)
   • The next host being in a susceptible state
   • The causative microorganism

7.

Medical Asepsis	Surgical Asepsis
a. Kills microorganisms on leaving the body	a. Kills microorganisms before entering body cavities
b. Clean technique with clean equipment and supplies	b. Sterile technique with sterile equipment and supplies
c. Used to prevent the transmission of microorganisms from person to another person	c. Used to maintain sterility when necessary to enter a sterile area of the body
d. Utilized during non-invasive procedures	d. Utilized for invasive procedures
e. Hands washed, or clean gloves on hands prior to handling any equipment or supplies	e. Hand washed with surgical scrub, sterile gloves worn to handle any equipment or supplies
f. Equipment and supplies are positioned are on clean field	f. Equipment and supplies are positioned on a sterile field
g. Protects both the health care professional and the patient	g. Protects the patient undergoing invasive procedures

8. Blood, blood products, human tissue, and body fluids to be considered as potentially infectious materials. In addition to blood and blood

products, semen and vaginal secretions, body fluids include cerebrospinal fluid, amniotic fluid, joint and other body cavity fluids, and nasal and oral secretions, including saliva.

9. Needlestick or sharps injuries must be reported after implementing first aid and cleansing procedures. The incident must be documented including a description of the incident (including date, time and place) and if possible identification of the individual whose body substance may have been on the contaminant. The employer has the responsibility to obtain consent to test the source's blood as soon as possible for HBV, HCV, and HIV. Some guidelines apply to source obtaining and testing blood refer to OSHA guidelines published by US Department of Labor. When test results are complete, the injured individual should be notified of the results within legal guidelines. The injured employee should sign consent allowing for testing of their blood as a baseline test. Follow-up testing should be performed within 90 days. If medically indicated, prophylaxis for post exposure should be provided to the employee.

10. The standards are to reduce employee exposure to the risk of infectious diseases such as hepatitis B virus (HBV) and human immunodeficiency virus (HIV) as they limit exposure.

CHAPTER 4

1. IV fluids are supplied in glass containers, semi-rigid plastic containers, and plastic containers called bags of fluids.
2. Glass containers are heavy, breakable and difficulty to store. Plastic containers are not breakable and are easier to store as well as being lighter in weight. Glass containers need venting and fluids are open to air because of this, while plastic bags are closed systems with less possibility of airborne contamination of fluids.
3. The major disadvantages of plastic containers are the inability to easily read the amount of fluid left in the container, the danger of leaks and tears to the containers, and the dangerous

interaction of plastic with medications that are used as additives.

4. The three types of major devices used to initiate IV infusions are needles—especially the scalp or winged needle, over the needle catheter and through the needle catheter.
5. Catheters, made of flexible plastic, are threaded through the lumen of the vein and the blunt tips on the catheters do not have the potential to cause the continued damage to the vein, as found with a needle. The use of a needle is for the short-term infusion. Also the catheter provides safety with the patient movement and ambulation. The catheter may be left in place for longer periods of time without the irritation to the vein walls.
6. Needleless systems, designed to prevent accidental needlestick injuries, are designed with blunt ends that pierce the ports on primary lines without the use of a needle. The port reseals with the removal of the needleless device.
7. The four most commonly used types of intravenous fluids are dextrose in water, sodium chloride (or saline) solutions, dextrose in saline, and Ringer's solutions.
8. Saline solutions are used to replace extracellular fluids lost through causes of dehydration and to correct water overload. They also replace sodium and chlorides that have been lost. Saline solutions are also used for diluent for medications that will be added to intravenous lines as well as being used to irrigate IV or intra-arterial devices.
9. Dextrose supplies calories for energy and to maintain homeostasis while sparing the use of body proteins. It provides the basic nutrition of sugars.
10. Pumps are more reliable for providing the patient with an accurate amount of fluids because the pump does not depend on gravity but rather uses pressure to infuse the fluids. This allows the resistance of external factors to be overcome. The pump has the ability to sense resistance and has alarms to indicate when the IV flow has been interrupted or other mechanical problems have occurred.

Other mechanical means such as clamps do not have the ability to overcome resistance because gravity is the means of infusion. Also, resistance from external forces may cause the discontinuation of the fluid infusion with the use of mechanical devices such as clamps.

CHAPTER 5

1. a. Kefurox 1.5 grams in 100 ml Dextrose 5% in normal saline to be infused over 1 hour IVPB using tubing of 10 drops/milliliter
   b. 33 gtts/min
   c. 1200 mg
   d. 53.3 or 53 ml
2. a. Furosemide 60 mg to be infused in 500 milliliters of Dextrose 5% in water using a drop factor of 20 drops/milliliter and 60 gtts per minute drip factor
   b. 272 minutes or 4.5 hours
   c. 0.2 mg/min
   d. 25000 mg
3. a. Add 60 units of Humulin-R to 100 milliliters of 2 1/2% Dextrose in 1/2 normal saline to be infused IVPB with a drop factor or 60 gtts/ml. The medication is to run at the rate of 2.5 U/ hour.
   b. 4.2 milliliters per hour
   c. 450 mg NaCl
   d. 2500 mg Dextrose
   e. 23.8 or 24 hours
   f. Humulin-R 0.6 ml
4. a. Add 1 gram Ampicillin sodium to 100 ml Lactated Ringer's to be infused over 2 hours using a drop factor of 60 drops/milliliter
   b. 100 ml/min
   c. 50 gtts/min
   d. 375 mg
5. a. Add 50 mg of Nitro-BID to 250 ml of Dextrose 5% in water to be infused at a rate of 5 micrograms per minutes using a drop factor of 60 drops/milliliter
   b. 20 mcg/ml
   c. 0.25 ml
   d. 300 min or 5 hours
   e. 25 milliliters

6. a. 3000 milliliters of Dextrose 5% in saline to be given on 24 hours using a drop factor of 15 drops/milliliter
   b. 1000 ml per 8 hours
   c. 3 containers
   d. 125 ml/hr
   d. 31 ml/min
   e. 625 ml
   f. 31.25 grams
7. a. 400 mg
   b. 8 ml
   c. 5 gtts/min
8. a. 33 min
   b. 3 containers of fluids
   c. 50 gm
   d. 100 gm
9. a. 0.69 or 0.7 ml/min
   b. 42 ml/hr
10. a. 1.5 ml/min in first hour
    b. 1.4 ml/min
    c. 510 ml in 6 hours
    d. 25 gm
    e. 4.5 gm

CHAPTER 6

1. The rationales or indications for using IV therapy fall into three categories: maintenance therapy, replacement therapy and restoration therapy.
2. Many factors things influence the normal intake of fluids, including the drinking of liquids, the consumption of food, and the oxidization of nutrients during metabolism.
3. Common medications that are administered intravenously include antimicrobial agents such as cephalosporins, aminoglycosides, penicillins; anticoagulants, antifungals, antiviral agents, bronchodilators, hypoglycemic drugs, insulin, immunosuppressants, biotherapy drugs, neuromuscular blocking agents, chemotherapy drugs and opioid drugs for intermittent or continuous pain relief.
4. Methods for the administration of medications or drug therapy include continuous or intermittent infusion, bolus injection, and piggy back infusion.

5. Individuals who are dehydrated; vomiting; experiencing electrolyte imbalance; unconscious; in shock; or unable to take medications, fluids, or nourishment orally benefit from the advantage of IV therapy as fluids and electrolytes are replaced. Additional advantages include the administration of antibiotics and other medications as many antibiotics require specific blood levels of their content to be maintained to reach optimum benefits. The requirement that blood levels remain constant to be effective is helped with IV therapy.

6. The patient complains of the skin will feeling tight and the skin appears stretched and taut. The signs are usually seen close to the insertion site including slowing or stopping of the fluid infusion, tissue induration, and swelling around the injection site with tissue remaining cool to touch.

7. The first line of defense of protecting the patient from infection as a result of IV therapy is the practice of good and consistent hand hygiene and proper medical asepsis.

8. Signs and symptoms of generalized infection include chills and fever, increasing heart and respiratory rate and dropping blood pressure. Anxiety and restlessness or lethargy are usually present. The patient may complain of not feeling "right" or advise "Something is wrong." These symptoms may be a delayed reaction after the IV has been discontinued.

9. In the early stages of fluid overload, the patient will display apprehension and some shortness of breath. Pulse, respiratory rates and blood pressure increase. As the amount of the overload increases, the patient may exhibit additional shortness of breath, anxiety, elevated blood pressure and a bounding pulse. Both respirations and pulse become more rapid. Edema is often present around the eyes and in the limbs, especially hands and ankles. Neck and limb veins appear distended. Skin appears taut and shiny and there may be peripheral cyanosis. Capillary refill is delayed and fluid is auscultated in the lungs. If possible to weigh the patient, a weight gain usually is

noted from before the onset of the therapy. Congestive heart failure and pulmonary edema are sequela that may be seen.

10. Symptoms and signs of pulmonary embolism are determined by the size and location of the embolism along with the general physical condition of the patient. Apprehension is common in these patients at the onset of the obstruction and during the course of treatment. The patient with a small, uncomplicated embolism experiences a cough, chest pain and low-grade fever. The patient with more extensive infarction will experience sudden onset of chest pain, acute shortness of breath, dyspnea and tachypenea with extreme anxiety. The heart rate will become very rapid and blood pressure drops significantly. This is caused by the migration of a clot from the limb to the pulmonary circulation where it becomes lodged in a smaller pulmonary vessel.

CHAPTER 7

1. The four processes of pharmacokinetics are absorption, distribution, metabolism, and excretion.

2. Absorption is not necessary in IV therapy because the medication is injected directly into the blood stream and does not have to be absorbed through the skin or intestinal tract.

3. Areas such as food and drug allergies, environmental factors, age, gender, lifestyles, amount of body fat, and preexisting conditions may be the answers used here. Other answers are possible.

4. A side effect is expected although undesirable in most cases. Adverse reactions are unexpected and can be life threatening such as anaphylaxis and severe drug allergies.

5. False. Absorption in the bloodstream is immediate with IV therapy because distribution throughout the body is almost immediate. Medications given intravenously cannot be retrieved nor the distribution in the

Appendix C   Answers to Review Questions   **145**

bloodstream stopped. This is one of the main dangers of IV administration of medications.

6. Anti-infectives, especially antibiotics, are the most frequently intravenously administered medications.

7. The main classifications of anti-infective medications given intravenously are antibiotics, antifungals, and antivirals.

8. The three dangers of prolonged use of anti-infectives are development of hypersensitivities, superinfections, and bacteria that become drug resistant to the medications.

9. Procaine penicillins should never be administered intravenously.

10. Most anti-fungals are in suspensions and in-line filters will remove any particles left in the fluids prior to reaching the blood stream.

11. By using veins from distal to proximal, the phlebitis will be distal to the possible areas for later venipunctures.

12. A bolus is a dose of IV medication given directly into a vein or tubing at a relatively rapid rate. An IV injection is given directly into the vein at a slower rate.

13. IV heparin may be given as a flush to retain patency of the IV lines during intermittent infusion or continuous infusion to prevent the formation of thrombi.

14. Total parenteral nutrition contains varying amounts of fats, proteins, carbohydrates, electrolytes, vitamins and minerals depending on the specific needs of the patient.

15. Peripheral parenteral nutrition, used for supplemental feedings, container fewer calories and less protein but problems such as phlebitis and infiltration into surrounding tissues are common problems. For prolonged use of TPN, a central catheter should be considered.

CHAPTER 8

1. Items to be checked before initiating IV therapy include patient's name, IV solution ordered to be administered, medication ordered to be added to the solution, amount of solution to be infused, time over which solution is to be infused or the time appropriate for the number of milliliters and any special instructions.

2. Signs to assess include presence of fever, presence of perspiration, dry warm skin, cracked lips, thirst, elasticity of skin, absence of moisture in axillae and/or concentrated, dark urine.

3. To prevent air bubbles from entering the bloodstream possibly resulting in an air embolism, air must be purged from the administration set tubing and any other tubing that may be attached to the set.

4. Drip chambers available include macro drip sets and micro drip sets. Macro drip chambers allow for the administration of 8 to 20 gtts per mL and micro drip sets allow for the administration of 50 to 60 gtts per mL.

5. Major factors to consider when selecting a vein to be used for an infusion site include a vein that is suitable size for a venipuncture device to be used to assure size to allow for amount of fluid to be infused; the type of fluid to be infused, especially the viscosity of the fluid; patient comfort and possible patient mobility. The condition, location and straightness of the vein should also be considered. The most distal acceptable site should be selected so that when more sites are required for venipunctures, it then is possible to move on up the arm to the larger veins closer to the heart since it is not possible to move back distally due to the fact that the lower veins that have been previously used should not be used again. Another factor to consider is avoiding veins over sharp bony areas or joints or veins in areas of recent trauma from injury or surgical procedures.

6. Methods used for compression above the site where a needle or catheter is to be inserted include having the patient clench his/her fist by opening and closing the fist to help pump blood into the vessels, helping them to distend; massaging the area in the direction of blood flow; applying a sphygmomanometer cuff on the limb above the intended site; inflating the pressure on the cuff just below systolic pressure; lightly and gently tapping the vein, being careful not to

injure the vein; allowing the limb to hang below the body placing it in a dependent position for a few minutes to distend the veins with blood; using a tourniquet or other means of constricting the vein above the intended site and applying moist heat to the area, often with a warm moist towel.

7. Hold the venipuncture device in the dominant hand while stretching the skin of the proposed site with the other hand stabilizing the vein. Hold the needle along side the vein with the bevel up at a 45° angle. Tell the patient that a sharp, quick stick will occur. Pierce the skin by inserting the needle distal and parallel to the vein at a 20 to 30° angle to the skin. Once the vein is entered, blood will flow back into the tubing or catheter hub. Slowly advance the needle into the vein approximately one inch and release the tension on the skin. Stabilize the needle or catheter with one hand and slowly release the tourniquet with the other hand. If the catheter is used, cover the stylet with the safety cap as it is removed. Keep the needle stable and dispose of the stylet in a rigid biohazard container.

8. The venipuncture site should be observed several times in the first thirty minutes and then at least hourly. The observation should include any signs of infiltration, leakage, bleeding, or potential infection. When the patient expresses feeling wetness around the dressing, or pain or tightness near the venipuncture site, the complaint should be immediately investigated by the clinician. The possibility of redness or abnormal warmth around the site should be observed and appropriate corrective measures taken. When infiltration is suspected and there is no blood return in the tubing when the container is lowered below the infusion site, the IV should be discontinued and restarted at a different location.

9. IV piggyback, bolus, and heparin or saline lock for IV injection.

10. The tubing is clamped shut and/or the infusion device is turned off, tape is loosened by the clinician and then the clinician applies gloves. A gauze pad is held in the non-dominant hand to be used to apply gentle pressure over the site as the needle or catheter is removed. The needle or catheter is gripped by the dominant hand and slowly withdrawn for the vein following the pathway of the vein and insertion. Pressure is held on the site until any bleeding ceases. A sterile dressing is applied to the site (often times a pressure dressing to apply gentle pressure over the site is required.) The patient is assessed for how the procedure was tolerated. Documentation of the discontinuation of the therapy is made along with a notation of any significant comments made by the patient. Documentation includes date, time, total amount and type of fluid infused, assessment of appearance of site and name or initials of clinician discontinuing the IV infusion. All materials are discarded according to OSHA guidelines with any sharps being placed in sharps containers and other materials properly disposed. The patient is assisted to area of dismissal, if appropriate.

Practice Problems

1. A physician orders a piggyback infusion containing Ampicillin in 75 mL of normal saline. The medication is to infuse over 1 hour using an infusion set of 50 gtt/mL.
   How many gtts/min will be infused?_____

2. A physician orders Oxytocin 10 units in 500 mL of NS to be infused over 30 minutes. The drop factor is 20 gtt/mL.
   How many gtts/min will be infused?_____
   How many units of Oxytocin will the patient receive in 20 minutes?_____

3. A physician orders Zantac 50 mg in 100 mL NS to infuse over 15 minutes. The drop factor is 15 gtts/mL.
   How many gtts/min will be infused?_____
   How many milligrams of Zantac will the patient receive in 10 minutes?_____

4. A physician orders Methylprednisolone succinate 500 mg in 150 mL NS to infuse over 2 hr. The drop factor is 20 gtt/mL.
   How many gtts/min will be infused?_____
   How many grams of NaCl are found in the fluids?_____
   If infused for 1 hour 15 minutes, how many grams of NaCl will be received by the patient?
   _____
   How many milligrams of the drug will be received in 1 hour 15 minutes?_____

5. A physician orders Nafcillin 1 g to be added to 100 mL D-5-W to run for 1 hour. The drop factor is 15 gtt/mL.
   How many gtt/min will be infused?_____
   How many milligrams of Nafcillin will be infused in 50 minutes?_____

6. A physician orders 2 L D-5-W to be infused at 25 gtts/min. The infusion set is 10 gtts/mL. What time is necessary for infusion of these fluids?_____

7. A physician orders Gentamycin 1.5 mg/kg/q8h IVPB in 150 mL NS for a patient who weighs 148 lb. The infusion is to be infused at 25 gtts/min. The drop factor is 20 gtts/mL.
   How many milligrams of Gentamycin should this patient receive?_____
   How long will it take for this medication to be infused in minutes?_____
   What total amount of Gentamycin will be infused daily?_____
   How many milligrams will the patient receive in 45 minutes?_____

8. A physician orders Oxacillin 12 g/day q3h IVPB in divided doses.
   How many milligrams of Oxacillin would be given to the patient with each dose?_____
   How many grams of Oxacillin would be given to the patient with each dose?_____
   If this comes in an IV infusion prepared from the following label, how many vials of Oxacillin would be necessary in 1 day?
   _____
   What would be the volume of medication to be added to NS 100 mL of fluids to fill this order?_____
   If the physician orders the medication to be given at 30 gtts/min and the drop factor is 20 gtts/mL, how long would this infusion take for completion?_____

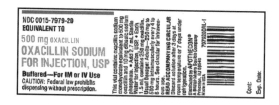

9. A physician orders the solution shown in the following illustration to be administered at 30 gtts/min using a drop factor of 50 gtts/mL.

How long will it take for this infusion to occur?_____

How many grams of Dextrose are in these fluids?_____

How many grams of sodium chloride are in these fluids?_____

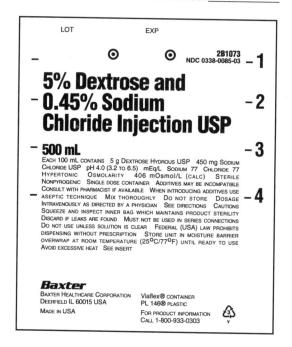

10. A physician orders Cefoperazone 2 g IV in LR 75 mL to be infused at 10 gtt/min. The drop factor is 25 gtts/mL.

How long will it take for the medication to infuse?_____

Using the following label, how many vials of Cefobid are required for this physician's order? _____

How many grams of Cefobid will be infused in 20 minutes?_____

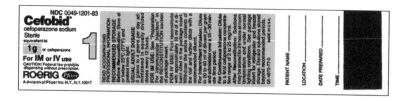

ANSWERS TO PRACTICE PROBLEMS

1. 63 gtts/min
2. 333 gtts/min; 7 (6.7) units
3. 100 gtts/min; 33 (33.3) mg
4. 25 gtts/min; 1.4 g; 0.9 (0.88) g; 313 (312.5) mg

5. 26 gtts/mL; 833 mg
6. 83 hr and 20 min
7. 101 mg; 2 hours; 303 mg; 38 mg
8. 1500 mg; 1.5 g; 24 vials; 9 mL; 1 hr and 13 min
9. 13 hours and 54 minutes; 25 g; 2.25 g
10. 3 hr and 8 min; 2 vials; 0.2 g

Index